POWERED
by HEALTH

The high-achieving
woman's guide to *health*,
vitality, and a new life full
of possibilities.

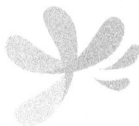

AMANDA BIGELOW

Published in Australia in 2015 by Amanda Bigelow

Banyo Qld 4014

Website: www.amandabigelow.com

National Library of Australia Cataloguing-in-Publication entry:

Bigelow, Amanda – author.

Powered by Health: the high-achieving woman's guide to health, vitality and a new life full of possibilities / by Amanda Bigelow.

9780994290106 (paperback)

Health

Well-being

Life skills

Women – Conduct of life

Self-actualization (Psychology)

613

Edited by Epiphany Editing & Publishing

Typesetting by Pipeline Design

Cover design by Pipeline Design

Printed in Australia by SOS Print + Media

CONTENTS

FOREWORD

This is what we've all been waiting for – an honest insight into health and wellbeing. How can we not have had this vision shown to us before? This book will act as your life guide – an almanac to living a life that is filled with inspiration and purpose. At a time where there's so much noise out there in the world of health, mindfulness and wellness, this book is likely to be all you need. It's not diets, nor fads, nor pills that will save us; it is pure knowledge and a better understanding of what affects our health that will enable us to enjoy happier and more fulfilled lives. Now is the time for every woman to think deeply about her health and wellbeing. With a holistic approach and an emphasis on moderation, I strongly believe this book will be the roadmap that all women have been waiting for.

This isn't just a book of insights and advice; it can also be used as a tool and guide to help you live a more wholesome lifestyle and to have a better understanding of yourself and your habits. It reminds us that health need not be complicated, but it does need to be integrated into our daily life. In order for our lives to really take shape in the way that we dream they can, we must consider all facets of our health and wellbeing – how everything affects our body as a whole and how we need to be ready to embrace the changes.

Amanda Bigelow invites us on a journey which encompasses a new way of considering and understanding health – nudging us away from the current trends and fads that are only bandaids for our problems. In the pages of her book, Amanda offers pragmatic and straightforward solutions and preventative measures for the many health problems we face in our stressful contemporary lives. As someone who has personally experienced my fair share of health issues since starting my own business, this book is a reminder for me to pay attention and delve further into my own wellbeing. It's something all of us have on our bucket list of things to do, yet somehow along the way we get distracted. As the well-known saying goes: 'It is only when we are sick that we realise what we should have done, and taking care of our health involves taking care of our mind, body and soul.'

To all of the high-achieving women out there, we must evolve and be courageous about our future. I recommend you read this book carefully and keep it somewhere easy to access so that it serves as a constant reminder of the importance of health and wellbeing. Refer to it whenever you need guidance; use it to nudge you into action every time you struggle or slip. Most importantly, let's all of us ensure that we pass on this knowledge to other women and help to spread the message of integrative health so that we all may benefit.

Grace Clapham

Co Founder of The Change School,
Change Ventur.es and Secret {W} Business,
and multiple award winning Changepreneur.

ACKNOWLEDGEMENTS

There are always a lot of people who help you along your journey every day and there are some people in particular who are dedicated to supporting you. I often look at trees or the sky or just people on the street and marvel at how wonderful life and the people in my life are. In saying that, I would especially like to acknowledge a few people here.

Huge thanks to Warren who has always believed in me and backed me for all I am worth.

My book mentor, Andrew Griffiths who supported and held me accountable for getting this book written. He is a champion.

My accountability buddies who have all been invaluable to this book publishing process. Everyone needs someone to hold them accountable.

My clients and colleagues who make all of my health discoveries real, and who so generously shared their stories for this book.

Grace Clapham who has supported me from the beginning of my business journey.

And perhaps oddly, but because it rings true for me, I want to acknowledge this place – our planet Earth – that enables us all to create and do meaningful things and share them with others.

PREFACE

Are you a high-achieving woman who is motivated to 'have it all' but finds it challenging to make this concept a reality? If so, it's quite likely that you know how important it is to be healthy in order to live an inspired and productive life.

Women are increasingly finding they are in a position to achieve their goals, whether they involve frequent travel; creating and growing a business; being of service to their community; taking on a promotion; juggling their work lives and looking after children; or just taking on the world. For women to handle all their activities in life, they need to be healthy, focused and balanced in all areas of their lives.

I know this fact from personal experience as I lost my health for a while and also lost my dreams. As a result of my high-achieving 'A' type personality, genetic predisposition, and life stress, I suffered two major health breakdowns and was forced to take stock of my health and my life.

Up until these health crises, my life had always been focused and goal oriented – my motto was work harder and harder. I took on impossible projects with great gusto and a mindset that I would succeed and solve any problem, no matter how challenging. And I did, but not without a huge toll on my health.

In my early career everything was fun and things were challenging, but also exciting. I took on more and more, until finally I became a corporate executive who ran and developed companies. I was working very long hours and frequently took work home.

Initially I became aware that my short-term memory was slipping and I often felt frazzled. I put work before exercise and I craved sugar. My weight had always yo-yoed and was an ongoing source of discontent and unhappiness – continually taking my focus away from enjoying life.

In my late forties, I was diagnosed with Hashimoto's Thyroiditis. I knew nothing about this disease or how to heal from it, and I soon learnt that Hashimoto's is a tricky disease to treat and to manage. My symptoms of joint pain, mood swings, and fatigue continued and I didn't know what to do. I sought help from chiropractors and doctors, and rested more. I kept up my usual diet of mostly healthy food, but still high in sugar and alcohol. Finally, I sought help from a naturopath and my health gradually improved over 12 months.

Feeling better again, I took on another exciting (yet highly stressful) career position. This point marked the start of my greatest downfall. After less than two years in this job, I had reverted to working relentlessly and my health problems returned with a vengeance. Finally, the crash came. I hit a wall of stress, insomnia, anxiety and productivity issues, and my world quickly tumbled around me. I became very depressed and was completely unable to cope.

First I became stressed, feeling as though I could never get everything done. This only fuelled the urge to work harder – after all, what else could I do to keep up? The presence of Hashimoto's made me more vulnerable to other conditions such as adrenal fatigue and weight gain. I became intensely focused on learning how to manage this debilitating disease with crazy symptoms that popped up in all different parts of my body.

The only thing that turned me around was a naturopath saying 'If you don't change your life you are headed for a train wreck.' It was at this point that I finally listened.

Finally I left my job and gradually healed over the following 18 months while, at the same time, experiencing total exhaustion, stress and anxiety, frequent crying spells, and panic about loss of income. There were many days when I wondered if I would ever recover, let alone work again.

Due to my health problems, I was forced to modify my 'A' type personality by learning to truly love my body and my mind, and to work with the essence of me – my spirit. I now live much more from my heart and am much less inclined to be dragged down by negativity and self-pity. I have come a long way – enough to say I love everything I do and I don't waste time doing anything I don't want to do. If I can pass on a thread – enough for you to take and develop into a wonderful tapestry of health and love – I will have fulfilled my purpose in writing this book.

Finally, I want to leave you with a story that has had a big impact on my life, and one that I hope will resonate with you on your own journey to finding true health.

Back in the late 1990s, I took a trip to the Canadian Arctic as part of a Winston Churchill Fellowship. I travelled as far as the tip of the landmass and then beyond to Banks Island, where the only natural herds of musk ox roam freely.

During my journey to the Arctic, I was fortunate enough to spend time with the local Inuit elders. I recall a rare encounter with Ruth, an Inuit elder in her late seventies who lived on a swiftly-flowing river that was home to a number of golden eagles.

It was mid-summer and she was busy preserving large amounts of wild salmon to tide her over the formidable winter months.

I sat down and watched her move with grace, energy, and purpose as she prepared the fish. I wondered how people could possibly live out the harsh winter months without daylight and in freezing conditions.

So I asked her how they managed to do this, and she told me something that deeply moved me. She said, 'We survive because we are fascinated with ourselves.'

I thought about what that meant for Ruth and her people, and I realised that they could never survive unless they had a close relationship with nature and the seasons. They recognised that they were part of nature and understood what they had to do in order to make it through each winter, during times when food was scarce.

Over the years, I came to understand that being fascinated with oneself is all about becoming curious and fully engaged with all that you can be.

For me, the idea behind Ruth's story now reminds me to be fully engaged in self-discovery in order to learn how to thrive in a high-pressure, increasingly toxic world. Self-discovery has driven me to understand the role of health in my life – how I can create my own version of a wonderful life and enjoy the feeling of coming home to myself. Now, it is my mission to help you and other women like you to achieve this in your lives as well.

Amanda Bigelow

INTRODUCTION

"FIND ECSTASY WITHIN YOURSELF.

IT IS NOT OUT THERE.

IT IS IN YOUR INNERMOST FLOWERING.

THE ONE YOU ARE LOOKING FOR IS YOU."

– OSHO

Women are incredible, fantastic and amazing. But most women I know don't acknowledge how special they really are. They do not look after themselves properly, and get caught up in the modern-day frenzy of tasks, duties and responsibilities. They are willing and present for everyone else but don't find time for themselves.

What happens to a woman's health and wellbeing if she spends most of her time looking after everyone else, and denies herself care and love? Ultimately, her health suffers; and the degree of suffering depends on her genetics, the amount of stress in her life, her diet, and her mental and physical wellbeing – her resilience.

In our busy lives, we constantly cross thresholds that put a great deal of pressure on our mind and body. To become fully healthy and to have the energy to live a fantastic life, we need to become more self-aware and nurturing toward ourselves. And just as important, is to understand that our health powers our vitality, productivity, and longevity.

Health and self-discovery are two important things that motivate me in all areas of my life. They help me to create positive outcomes, understand myself, and live through my core values. For me, health is a holistic concept which involves eating well and doing what nourishes my body and my mind. Self-discovery helps me to become attuned to those changes in me and in my world that will bring me the results I'm seeking in my life. I love to imagine how my life will be transformed when I reach a particular goal. As a health coach and behavior change specialist, my objective is to share my experience with you and help you to discover true health and wellbeing for yourself.

If I were to sum up the benefits of health and self-discovery, I would say that together they form two matching golden keys that enable you to learn and grow, and to be and do all the things you want in life. Through good health, you can physically and mentally keep up with life. From self-discovery, you gain self-awareness, motivation, and greater interest in life. You develop a deeper understanding of other people, and you become far more resourceful because you have more knowledge and wisdom.

My motivation for writing this book is to provide a clear pathway that will lead you to boundless energy, lasting vitality, a renewed body and, ultimately, to a life where you feel that you are powered by health. Based on the Five Principles of Integrative Health which I teach to my clients (and practise myself), my desire is to open the door to a world of endless possibilities and for you to feel as though you've finally 'come home'.

Feels Like Home

Think about the term 'home' for a minute. What comes to mind? Is your idea of home the house that you so lovingly renovated, the smile on your child's face, your dribbling, deliriously happy dog who greets you at the end of a long work day? Or is it that feeling you get when you curl up on the sofa with a hot chocolate and a great book? It's such a wonderful sensation to feel at home.

What if you could feel a permanent, unwavering sense of home that belonged to you and you alone; that did not rely on an attachment to people, places, things and events? This kind of home dwells within you and is available to you all of the time. It comes when you find the interest and courage to pursue health in all areas of your life. It is like a deep stillness within you that you can always reach into and readily use in your life.

In this place called 'home' you are permanently aligned with yourself. Sure, you will have moments when you lose yourself, but you will have the roadmap to get you back on track. You will make informed choices about all aspects of your life, and you will know whether your decisions will nourish you or have the opposite effect.

Over the last few decades, the world has undergone dramatic changes. Work has become progressively more stressful and demanding; people's material expectations have risen dramatically; self-doubt, anxiety, stress, and depression are all on the rise; and the feeling that we have to be everything to everybody has become the norm. The world is now full of continual media coverage, influence from self-interested multi-national corporations, constant entertainment, and the proliferation of negative news. As a result, we are becoming increasingly disconnected from ourselves as we constantly respond to external stimuli and huge volumes of information that invade us.

What would the benefits be if you were able to find a level of stillness and strength within you that enabled you to deal with the expectations and challenges of life today?

In a recent interview, body-mind-spirit nutritionist Dr. Deana Minich expressed it well when she said that in relation to complete health, there are three questions we need to ask ourselves:

1. What do we avoid?

2. What nourishes us?

3. What makes us thrive?[1]

Health happens when you are in harmony with all parts of yourself. It happens because the act of connecting aligns all facets of who you are. As a result, you value all of you and you want to love your body, look after it, treasure it, make it happy, and be in harmony with it.

Reconnecting with yourself is a deliberate, conscious decision to change your health and your life for the better – and for the long term. The prize is what happens as a result of committing to that life-changing journey: you come home to yourself.

This process often comes after a health crisis or major event in your life that wakes you up to your previous poor lifestyle choices and decisions. You arrive at a crossroads and are forced to look at your life habits and behaviour addictions. In practical terms, reconnecting with yourself comes in parts – all of your parts and all of your life.

This book is based on my Five Principles of Integrative Health, and will show you how to apply each in your life. These five principles are:

- your body – nutrition and fitness

- your mindset

- your spiritual wellbeing

- your work and career

- your relationships.

I have included two 'bookend' concepts to enable you to achieve and maintain health in these areas: at the start I cover the actions necessary to establish your health intentions and goals, and I close by asking you to reflect and maintain your new life.

Part One: Establishing Your Health Intentions and Goals

The journey starts with establishing your intentions and goals for your health and life. It is really important to fully understand why you want to pursue better health and a new life. When you write down your goals and intentions, tell others about them, and start to live them. Now you are on the path to better health and wellbeing.

Part Two: Your Body – Nutrition and Fitness

In this section, I discuss the principle of nutrition and fitness, and explore what nourishes your body so you can tune into what foods and movement your body thrives on. Your body is highly intelligent, and if you work with it and trust that it has the innate wisdom to know what is best for you, it will be able to heal itself. Learning about what your body needs to thrive, and then acting upon that knowledge, is the single best thing you can do to lay down the foundations of food/body connection for the rest of your life.

We all want our body to be fit and look great. We want to feel beautiful, inside and out.

'And so you shall,' said the fairy godmother. But I am not your fairy godmother and it is not fantasy that exercise will result in a healthy, lean, and active body. So why is it that we don't like to exercise or cannot seem to make it a natural part of our lives? Maybe it is because we are doing the wrong kind of exercise for our body? Or maybe we don't like exercise and are just going through the motions? In this part, we will examine the on/off exercise routine and we will find the right movement for your body – movement that works for you and your lifestyle.

Part Three: Your Mindset

Here we move on to the more challenging aspect of our lives – the habits, emotions, and mental addictions that keep us acting against our body, mind, and spirit. If we are facing a crossroads in our health, there will be attitudes that have contributed to our health problems. This section focuses on making real health breakthroughs in our life and achieving clarity of mind in order to make decisions that will nourish us.

Part Four: Your Spiritual Wellbeing

This is the bridge to take you beyond the health and fitness regime that you have been incorporating into your life. It is designed to reconnect you with nature in simple daily ways, as well as help you become grounded in your changes and develop a deeper self-awareness. From this point, the pathway is becoming much clearer; your mind, body, and spirit are beginning to soar like an eagle.

Part Five: Your Work and Career

With your deepening perspective on what nourishes your life, you will be ready to examine the work you do and determine whether or not it really brings you satisfaction and happiness every day – or at least most days. Is there a niggling, reoccurring voice in your head that tells you there must be more? This section explores how you can make decisions and changes in your career in order to enable you to really shine.

Part Six: Your Relationships

Looking at all of your significant relationships – good and not so good – is like peeling open a sardine tin. This is possibly the hardest aspect of your health to review and change. But don't worry: you can start at a point where you feel comfortable. I will show you a way to see relationships in an entirely different light: a way that takes the fear of conflict and the fear of change out of improving your relationships, and demonstrates how to cut ties with those people that don't nourish you.

Part Seven: Reflecting on Your New Life

This final section is where you start to put it all together – to review and examine how far you have come in your life. Maybe you only attempted some of the activities in a few sections of this book and felt that was all you required. Maybe you wandered through it, picking out those chapters that seemed to be most interesting or relevant to you. It is important that you take from this book what best suits you as an individual. The crucial thing is to reflect on your new and improved life.

Replace the cliché that we live in rapidly changing times with the awareness that you can find ways to thrive rather than just survive amidst the pressures of life today.

I recommend that you work through my Five Principles of Integrative Health – not necessarily in order – and that you apply and imbibe the important aspects of them in your life. Once you get a taste of renewed energy and vitality, you will find that this lifestyle becomes your preferred way of living.

Someone once said to me, 'People who do things, get things'. It is my pledge to you that if you do the 'integrative health thing', you will end up with the results you dream of.

Five principles of Integrative Nutrition

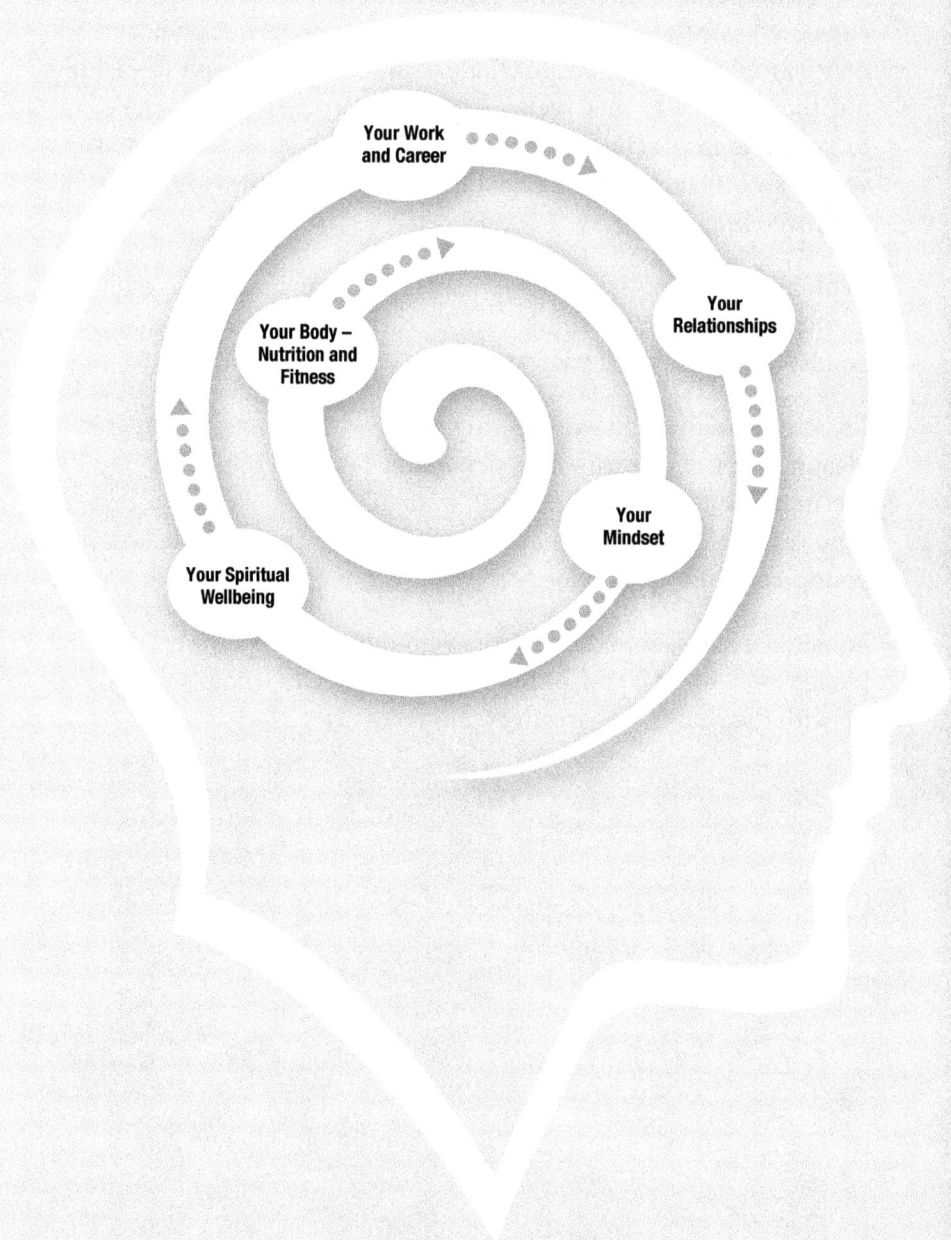

Your Work and Career

Your Relationships

Your Body – Nutrition and Fitness

Your Mindset

Your Spiritual Wellbeing

PART ONE

Establishing Your Health Intentions and Goals

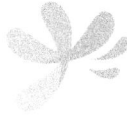

Chapter 1
The Journey of Integrative Health

The concept and practice of integrative health is a revolutionary way of approaching health and wellness, where health is related to the whole – body, mind and lifestyle. For example, poor nutrition, stress, insomnia, lack of exercise, career dissatisfaction and toxic relationships all have a negative impact on our health and wellbeing. If you want to be completely healthy and prevent illness, you need to look after all areas of your life. Solving a nutritional problem by changing the food you eat is often the first step, and while an important part of your health, it is only one aspect. You need to look after all parts of your being if you want to be truly healthy.

The three main problems I find high-achieving women commonly face today are:

- Low energy
- Excess weight
- Stressed and feeling stuck

Often these are the signs that women will notice first. They are important health indicators as they can be the precursors for other chronic illnesses such as autoimmune diseases and serious digestive conditions. With 21st Century lifestyles placing so much pressure on our bodies, and the stress of modern living and keeping up taking its toll, there has also been a huge increase in food sensitivities, sleep deprivation, and sugar in people's diets.

Yet, the majority of chronic illnesses, also (or what are termed 'lifestyle diseases') can be prevented.

We need a different response to individual and community health today. We need a response that addresses the cause of our symptoms. Integrative health is the perfect solution to the many stressful physical, mental and psychic forces that have a negative impact on our lives. It just makes good sense to delve into all areas of our lives in order to heal them.

The Five Principles of Integrative Health

Your Body – Nutrition and Fitness

Our body is the physical vehicle that carries us through life. In this way, our body is our temple that should be loved and nourished so that it, in turn, can look after us for a long time. Our body is where we develop the many physical symptoms and ailments that can occur through a combination of circumstances such as genetics, poor self-care, stress, environment and lifestyle. When people want to become healthy, they usually work on their body first. On the whole, eating healthy food and exercising tends to be the main focus in our society today.

Physical health is very important, but is only one part of the story that leads to complete health. We now know that mindset and other parts of our life play a huge role in determining our health and wellbeing. In fact, in many instances, mindset is more important than nutrition.

Your Mindset

Up until only a few years ago, mental health in Australia was a term used in reference to mental illness. Now it has a broader meaning and includes clinical and non-clinical mental health. In my opinion and experience, the mind and emotions are amongst the greatest contributing forces to both great health and poor health. I often find that I start out working with my female clients around weight loss and then we delve into the real issues, which are mindset and negative thinking patterns that prevent them from becoming healthy and vital. In addition, many conditions such as anxiety and depression can improve with the right nutrition, and with a diet that focuses on healing the gut and intestinal microbiome. Recent research indicates that the health of the gut has the capacity to influence the immune and endocrine systems which form a communication pathway between the microbiota and brain health and disease. This is known as the microbiome-brain-gut axis.[2]

Your Spiritual Wellbeing

Your spirit is your momentum in life: the light or spark within you that gets you up every morning. A close relationship with your own spirit along with engaging your own form of spirituality can really support your resilience and your health. I include nature here because it can be a great teacher. It is mine and always has been. We are all part of nature but often we live as though we are not. This early part of the 21st Century is a time for you to make sure you don't through away what makes you human – nature included.

Your Work and Career

Work can give a great sense of accomplishment and joy, or it can be the source of discontent and stress in life. Too often we can lose our perspective about what our work is meant to be. We view it as a source of income rather than a source of inspiration and contribution. This is an important area to examine in regard to our health and wellbeing.

Your Relationships

Relationships of all kinds can have a huge impact on your health. If you find yourself trapped in a toxic relationship your health will suffer. I think we can do better in our relationships by developing the courage to improve them or let them go. If we are going to be truly healthy, we would do well to clean up our own behaviour, as well as recognise those relationships that do not nourish us.

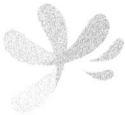

SIMPLE GUIDELINES FOR IMPROVING YOUR HEALTH

If your energy is flagging and you feel tired on a daily basis, the following suggestions will help you to feel better and improve your health:

1. Test yourself for gluten and dairy intolerances by eliminating them both from your diet for one to two weeks and observing any changes. Read my instructions on Chapter 4 for advice about how to do this.

2. Eat more vegetables daily. Load your plate with a rainbow of vegetables, along with some protein, grains and fats.

3. Get 7 – 8 hours of sleep per night.

4. Drink at least 8 glasses of water each day.

5. Crowd out sugar by replacing it with healthy snacks.

6. Reduce your intake of processed foods. Instead, focus on eating whole foods as much as possible.

7. Find a way of exercising that you love; not one that is pushed at you by the media or through peer pressure. Everything you do for yourself should be about enjoyment not regiment.

8. Spend time in nature where you can reflect and contemplate your goals and approaches to life.

9. Keep a journal to help you identify the toxic or negative self-talk in your life.

10. Venture out and try some new activities that nourish your spirit.

11. Take a close look at your relationships. It can be difficult to do, but, as with everything else in your life, take it step-by-step. Remember that in order to create a new life with different possibilities, your changes will bring forward new people with whom you can share new experiences. Some of your old relationships will fall away naturally as you create new colleagues, friends and opportunities.

12. Work on the Five Principles of Integrative Health in your own time to make step-by-step changes that nourish your health and your life.

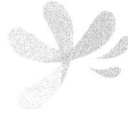

Chapter 2
Setting Your Personal Intentions and Goals

Before embarking on your journey to better health and wellbeing, it's vital for you to decide on your personal intentions and goals so that you know where you are heading.

Your Intentions

Setting your intentions is about identifying why you want to have a healthy and productive life for many years to come. If you identify the 'why' and have a very clear picture in mind, you will have a much greater chance of following through and making your health goals a reality.

Some of the reasons why you might want to improve your health could include:

- living well for many years with low morbidity
- getting more things happening in your life
- having more energy and vitality to enjoy life
- slowing down the aging process
- keeping up with your kids
- avoiding serious illness
- being highly productive throughout all your life.

The following exercise will help you identify your health intentions. Keep in mind that many small steps will lead to big results. Once you start to develop a close relationship with your body, mind and spirit, your life will become clearer, more joyful and more aligned to those times when you were at your best.

- In a journal or safe place write down everything that sums up why you are reading this book and why you want to improve your health. Think about how things are for you now, and how you would like them to be in the future. Now, write down all the reasons why you want to do this.

- You may also like to draw a symbol or an image that encapsulates your reasons for seeking better health. Take time to do this – enjoy the process, play some inspiring music while you draw, make it colorful. The important thing is to put your energy into the drawing.

Once you have finished, focus your mind on the drawing and the words. Place one or both items somewhere prominent where you will see them daily. This will help to motivate you to make a regular commitment to your health and wellbeing.

Your Goals

Setting and working with goals is a fundamental step in the journey to achieving what you want in your health and in your life. I have worked with goals all of my life. Generally, I write them down, print them out and then stick the page on the wall in my office. I want to be able to look at them, feel them and know them. When I have achieved these goals, I am then motivated to set more.

I have also learnt not to have too many goals at the same time. Make goals for the big things in your life that really matter to you. The small things often get in the way of big goals, so watch out they don't take over. Use your 'to do' list or your calendar to deal effectively with daily goals or tasks. The small goals should reflect your bigger ones. You can also invest in an organisation application such as MyLifeOrganised (MLO). There are plenty to choose from online.

The easiest way to identify and feel aligned with your goals is to start out with medium-term goals and chunk them down into shorter-term goals. I like to set annual, quarterly, and monthly goals in that order. I also have 20-year goals that are not so specific but are my guiding lights. I set them for my health, my work, my social life and my personal development.

Goals are interesting and not as dry as you might think. Have some fun with them, treasure them and celebrate them when you reach them, no matter how big or small they are.

The act of setting a goal is a process, not a rigid procedure that you stick to. For example, I set monthly goals and then often find that they need to be changed. This might be because I realised that my original goal wasn't exactly what I wanted or sometimes I learnt something new and the goal was no longer relevant.

When you set your own goals, remember that it is a flexible process that not only drives you to reach your goals, but allows you to go deeper and find new and different goals.

Goals are best when they are specific. Make them clear and measurable. Let's say you want to lose weight. Start with identifying what your ideal weight is and set a timeframe to achieve this goal by. For example: if you decide that you want to lose five kilos over six weeks, you could set a halfway mark of 2.5 kilos in three weeks. At this point, you could celebrate your success with a massage or something that nourishes you and motivates you to keep going.

Here is my recommended framework for setting goals in your life, along with some examples:

Set three annual goals

- Develop a healthy exercise and movement way of life that is fun, consistent, and fits in with my lifestyle. This includes walking regularly, yoga, and playing tennis.

- Find my true purpose and passion in life. Review my current work and investigate new ideas for a career change.

- Improve my overall diet and lose weight slowly and surely. I will aim to lose 20 kilos within 12 months.

Set three quarterly goals

Notice that these goals are stated as though they have already been achieved. This works as well.

- I am walking two times a week for 40 minutes, attending two yoga classes a week and playing tennis once a week

- I am clear about what my purpose in life is.

- I have lost seven kilos and have gone down one dress size.

Set monthly goals

- I am walking three times a week for 30 minutes. I am also doing yoga once a week and have found a partner to play tennis with.

- I have bought and read a book on finding my life's purpose and I have taken notes. I am writing daily about what I feel it might be.

- I have lost three kilos and am noticing that my clothes are now looser.

I hope these examples provide you with some inspiration. Remember, the only rules are to make your goals specific and measurable. You can write them in the way that works best for you – present tense or future tense. Don't get hung up on perfecting them. The key is get going and start implementing them. You will build momentum as you achieve them. The trick is to do them, track them, celebrate them when you've achieved them, and then happily set some more.

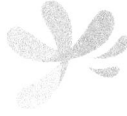

Chapter 3
Reviewing Your Current Health Status

How healthy are you? If you are a high-achieving woman, it makes sense that having great health and vitality will power a high level of productivity and enable you to accomplish all the amazing things you want in your life. If you have already experienced a few health issues, then now is the time to establish good health principles so you are constantly powered by wellbeing, great food and lots of fun.

How does your health rate in an integrative health model?

Do you eat reasonably healthily but still regularly have to cope with issues such as mood swings? Do you have low energy at certain times of the day? Are you struggling to get the right amount of sleep? Do you find it challenging to find time to cook healthy meals?

Most of us experience lifestyle tensions such as problems at work or relationship issues. But often we don't realise that when we are not in harmony with our lives, we are not in harmony with ourselves. As a result, we can become physically and mentally unwell.

I have created a simple survey for you to take that provides you with an indication of where you are in terms of your health. The survey is designed to give you an overall understanding of your level of health within the integrative health spectrum.

Feels Like Home Health Survey

Survey Questions		Tick for yes
Nutrition & Digestion		
1	Do you eat out more than two or three times per week?	
2	Are your meals and snacks more than 20 per cent processed foods?	
3	Do you eat more than 5–6 teaspoons of sugar on a daily basis?	
4	Does your meal mostly consist of pasta, grains, or meat, and few vegetables?	
5	Are you carrying more weight than you would ideally like to?	
6	Is you energy low after meals (especially lunch)?	
7	Do you feel bloated or get gas after eating?	
8	Do you have less than one daily bowel movement?	
9	Do you suffer from constipation or bouts of diarrhea?	
10	Do you wake up in the morning feeling tired and worn out?	

| 11 | Have you taken a course of antibiotics recently or several times throughout your life? | |
| 12 | Have you recently spent time in developing countries where you contracted a bug, virus, or other pathogen? | |

If you ticked the majority of the boxes above, it is likely that you may be experiencing some type of digestive problem that requires attention. If you ticked number 12, you may need to have some tests done to find out if you still have a pathogen or bug in your gut.

Exercise & Movement

1	Do you do struggle to fit exercise or regular movement into your week?	
2	Do you start an exercise program and then give up?	
3	Is finding time to get regular exercise difficult for you?	
4	Do you find exercise a chore?	
5	Do you have trouble getting to sleep or do you wake up during the night and struggle to get back to sleep?	
6	Do you have sufficient energy to get through the day without feeling tired?	

If you ticked four out of six boxes, you may need to reassess your work and life commitments to allow you enough time and energy to exercise. It may also be that you are not doing the sort of exercise that you love. Finding the right mix that you will enjoy could be what you need.

Mindset

1	Do you find that all the enjoyable things you want to do in your life always get put on the backburner?
2	Think about how positive or negative you regularly feel. Would you say, on balance, that you are more negative than positive?
3	Do you experience mood swings often?
4	Are you lacking in self-confidence?
5	Do you suffer from anxiety, excessive stress, or do you worry a lot?
6	Do you have depression or have you had it previously?
7	Do you feel that life is not much fun anymore?

If you ticked three or more boxes, you are likely to be 'stuck' and experiencing some mindset and emotional issues in your life. If you ticked numbers 5 and 6, you might want to see a professional practitioner to help you deal with these issues. You might also like to ask your doctor or health professional to undertake a test to check for Vitamin D deficiency. This can be a common cause of mood issues, as this vitamin is very important for your overall health and emotional wellbeing.

Spirit

1	Have you been feeling that you are unsure of your purpose in life?
2	Do you find it difficult to take time out, contemplate your life and feel recharged and renewed?
3	Do you spend a lot of time watching television, the news and staying indoors?

4	Do you find that you get up daily and feel that you are just going through the motions of life?	
5	Does the idea of yoga, meditation, or silence turn you off?	
6	Are you lacking confidence in your work and personal life?	
7	Is spirituality unappealing to you?	
8	Do you find that you often feel flat and bored with life?	

If you ticked four or more boxes, then finding some purpose and meaning in your life could help awaken you to increased opportunities. Also, you might find reading some thoughtful books, walking in nature, or getting involved with some new hobby or activity very beneficial.

Work

1	Do you stay back at work late on a regular basis?	
2	Do you take work home and work late into the night?	
3	Are you unhappy with your work or workplace?	
4	Do you wake up in the morning and dread the idea of going to work?	
5	Do you have few hobbies and interests other than work?	

If you ticked three or more boxes you need to reassess your work and lifestyle choices. Look at how much work you are currently doing and if it is time for a change.

Relationships

1	Do you have repetitive thoughts that significant relationships in your life (such as with your family and/or partner) are not working well?	
2	Are you unsure of the value of your other significant relationships?	
3	Are you a loner and someone who has very few or no real friends?	
4	Do you have problems with any of your siblings that often trouble you and you don't know how to solve?	
5	Do you have any significant issues with people at your work place that have a detrimental impact on your job or role?	
6	Are there any people in your life you would like to let go of but don't know how?	

If you ticked three or more boxes, it is probably time to examine some of your relationships in your life. You may want to seek professional support to help you find an effective way of dealing with them.

Your survey results

If you answered the survey above with more ticks/yeses than blanks in each table then you do need to think about these important areas in your life and what you could do (no matter how small) to tackle some of these problems.

This survey is not intended to be a thorough examination of your health habits and history; it is designed to be more of an indication for you. However, it does offer you an overall method for discovering certain things in your life that you might need to work on or get further tests for.

For the most part, you can use this survey to make adjustments where your scores indicate that action is required. If you have any doubts or have any major concerns after doing this survey, be sure to seek advice from your doctor or health professional.

Remember, we are all human and so all of us have areas in our lives that need to be addressed. If we didn't, we wouldn't be human!

Having great health is about taking back your power and assuming responsibility in all areas of your life. It's about tuning in over time and learning to listen to all of the parts of you. It's about ensuring that you are getting the right nutrition the majority of the time.

As your health journey progresses, you will naturally find that your diet and life becomes more energised and more peaceful. You may find that you are eating fewer processed foods, drinking less, exercising regularly, and getting more sleep. This is mostly how it goes. It really is quite easy and straightforward when you follow a few guidelines and make some simple choices.

PART TWO

Your Body –
Nutrition and Fitness

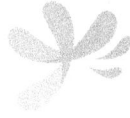

Chapter 4
Understanding What Nourishes Your Body

"THE FOOD THAT YOU EAT CAN BE EITHER

THE SAFEST AND MOST POWERFUL

MEDICINE OR, THE SLOWEST FORM OF POISON."

– ANN WIGMORE

Be your own Detective

When I work one-on-one with high-achieving women the first thing I do is to find out 'what is going on inside'. This involves detective work and is the foundation for designing a wellness program to help my clients heal and nourish their bodies. We work on this process together, and importantly, I teach them how to investigate and learn what is right for them as individuals.

I want you to be your own detective with the skills, over time, to know what is going on in your body and your life, and then to take action. As you get to know your body much better you will learn what foods it thrives on, and which foods either harm it or just don't nourish it. Doing this is a huge step forward in your ability to look after your health.

Of course, you will still need doctors, physicians and health practitioners. This is not intended to replace them. It is simply designed to help you know how to look after your own body and to work with health professionals when necessary.

Have you heard of the term 'functional nutrition' or 'food as medicine'? It is becoming increasingly popular today. Most people are adopting aspects of it through eating some (or all) of the different available 'super foods'.

However, functional nutrition involves more than super foods; it's about knowing what is right for your body. For example, kale was the big new thing a while ago, but raw kale in a smoothie can be harsh and not nourishing for people who have digestive issues. Lightly steamed kale is fine. So there are some instances where raw foods are not good for certain people. Another example is the nightshade family of vegetables; the main ones being potatoes, tomatoes, bell peppers and eggplants. For some people, especially those with arthritis, joint pain, gastroesophageal reflux disease (or GERD), or other digestive issues, vegetables belonging to the nightshade family can cause or exacerbate these conditions because they are allergic (or have a sensitivity) to them.[3]

These are a few examples which demonstrate that our health can be greatly helped by knowing more about our bodies and what works best for us.

Become your own health detective and find out if you have food sensitivities or allergies.

Crossing Thresholds

There are so many new dietary theories, programs, and answers available now. In my opinion, this trend is both very exciting and confusing at times. Vegetarian, paleo, omnivore, pescatarian, vegan, raw food, organic, fruitarian, anti-inflammatory diet, zone diet, five/two diet, gluten-free, dairy-free, and so on – there is a seemingly endless list of current diet theories and eating practices. It's exciting because we are all starting to understand and define our differences, and now we can eat at home and in restaurants according to our preferences.

I am an omnivore and I eat a diversity of foods that is proportionally balanced between vegetables, complex carbohydrates, lean protein, good oils and fats, fresh herbs and spices, and clean water. I tend to follow an anti-inflammatory, gluten and dairy free diet. I rarely eat processed foods, and I favour mostly organic seasonal, local, whole foods. I have designed this way of living through experimentation and keeping a food/mood journal to tell me how my body responds to certain foods. My diet considers the environment and I include mostly local and seasonal foods that are organic.

I also live by the 80/20 rule of eating: to maintain my body's optimum health, I eat healthy for 80 per cent of the time and the other 20 per cent I eat whatever I want. Generally speaking, this means that I still eat mostly healthy foods because, over time, my tastes and cravings have changed from eating a lot of sugar to eating more nourishing foods. This is the wonderful aspect of treating health and wellness as a journey.

I also like to do an annual detox to help my liver and gut stay in top condition.

I believe it is easy to make a dogma out of anything, and that includes food. If we become overly fixated on our diet, it tends to rule us and we box ourselves into a life without enjoyment; always thinking about how we have to eat versus how we can eat. (The exception, of course, is people with health issues that require specific dietary control).

It is important to follow a nutritional path that is currently backed by sound research, and is one that your body loves because it is being nourished by the foods you are providing for it.

The Food/Mood Journal

I ask all new clients to keep a food/mood journal for a week. Recording what you eat and how you feel afterwards will reveal any major food intolerances such as gluten and dairy – the two most obvious ones. If you are starting your health journey, I highly recommend that you keep a food/mood journal for seven days.

The most common symptoms of food intolerances are listed below.

For gluten:

- Bloating
- Gas
- Irritable bowel (IBS) or constipation
- Headaches
- Brain fog
- Swelling and pain in joints
- Mood swings
- Nausea

For dairy:

- Sinus and mucus issues
- Gas
- Diarrhea or loose stools
- Gurgling or rumbling in stomach
- Cramps in lower intestines

After you have finished recording your daily food intake for a week and have analysed your food/mood journal for correlations to any symptoms, all you need to do is to remove gluten and dairy items from your diet and observe how you feel from there on. If your symptoms disappear, you would do well to exclude gluten from your food. You could try reintroducing dairy, but if the symptoms come back, exclude dairy foods as well.

Gluten from wheat, barley and rye is present in breads, cakes, pasta, biscuits and other foods. It is also in many processed foods, such as soy sauces, ice cream and other foods. This tends to trip people up unless they are vigilant about reading food packaging labels.

Gluten and dairy are the two big culprits in people's diets, causing increases in food sensitivities and intolerances in many individuals, ranging from mild sensitivity to high sensitivity, and to Celiac disease, which is very serious.

If you think that sensitivity to gluten may be an issue in your diet, I recommend you refer to the following website: www.thedr.com. Dr Tom O'Bryan (based in the USA) specialises in gluten intolerance and is also very well informed about other food intolerances.

Fortunately, because so many of us are sensitive to gluten and cannot digest it properly, following a gluten-free diet is not such a drama in

Australia. There are many gluten-free products available on the market, and many restaurants these days cater for gluten and dairy-free diets.

In addition to gluten and dairy, there are others foods and substances that can cause problems. If you don't feel better after removing gluten and dairy, I suggest you get a series of food sensitivity/allergy tests done by your doctor. Alternatively, you can try the elimination diet which is much more restrictive and useful for people who are feeling really unwell.

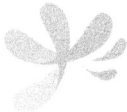

FOOD SENSITIVITIES AND INTOLERANCES - ANNE'S STORY

Anne had reached a point in her health journey where she was eating well, but she often felt bloated, nauseous, and suffered from other digestion issues. She had a number of tests done that showed her she was intolerant to gluten and lactose. So Anne had to face the idea of cutting gluten and lactose out of her diet. This meant eliminating wheat, rye and barley products which includes bread, pasta, biscuits, cakes and a variety of sauces and condiments such as soy sauce and even vegemite. In addition, Anne needed to cut out milk, cheese of all kinds, ice cream, cream and all other dairy products.

This presented Anne with a difficult situation as previously she'd been able to eat whatever she'd wanted. Now, all of sudden, she had to cut out half of the foods she'd regularly eaten. The way that Anne tackled this dilemma was to find out how she could replace the items she could no longer eat. She discovered a lot of gluten-free products including bread and pasta in her supermarket, and she also minimised her lactose intake. She tried lactose-free milk and found it too sweet, and then she tried rice and almond milk, as well as coconut milk and cream and coconut butter which she quite enjoyed.

Initially, Anne concentrated on removing gluten and dairy from her diet, but her first choice was to still include the alternatives in the types of processed foods she'd always enjoyed. The problem was that many commercially produced gluten-free products contain other substances like sugar and preservatives that are not healthy either.

Once Anne had become used to removing gluten and dairy foods from her diet, the next step was to find great recipes and to experiment with cooking whole foods that are gluten and dairy free. Coconut products now formed a larger component of her diet. She successfully crowded out processed gluten and dairy products from her life and shifted her diet to to more healthy foods overall.

Due to growing numbers of people like Anne discovering that they need to modify their diet for the sake of their health, restaurants are responding by creating delicious, healthy meals free of gluten, sugar and dairy.

As a result of changing her diet by making step-by-step adjustments, Anne found that her life was better and she felt healthier and had renewed energy.

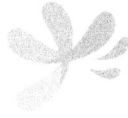

Chapter 5
Boosting Your Nutritional Levels

So, having made the decision to begin your journey to better health, what can you do to boost your nutritional levels? The trick to shifting your diet to a healthy one without creating a major upheaval in your life is to do it step by step; making a few changes here and there that are easy to incorporate into your daily routine.

Here are my top seven steps to help you to easily improve your nutrition.

Eat more vegetables and balance your plate

Most of us don't eat enough vegetables. To get more energy in your life, I recommend that you aim to have 50 per cent veggies on your plate, 25 per cent protein and 25 per cent carbohydrate. It's a good idea to have a diversity of vegetables on your plate, like a 'rainbow' – red, green, orange, purple veggies and so on. Different colours mean that you have a range of vitamins and minerals in your diet to energise your body.

Go for greens

Despite the 'green smoothie revolution', greens are often the most important vegetable missing in our diets. Including dark leafy greens in your list of daily foods is essential to establishing a really healthy body and robust immune system. Another really important role green vegetables play is to balance the pH levels in your body. Green vegetables are high alkaline foods. Our bodies thrive in an alkaline condition and can become disease-ridden in an acidic body.

Here are some of the main benefits of green vegetables:

- blood purification
- cancer prevention
- improved circulation
- strengthened immune system
- improved liver, gall bladder, and kidney function
- promotion of intestinal flora (or what is now known as our intestinal microbiome).

My suggested list of green vegetables for you to include regularly in your diet includes:

kale, broccoli, bok choy, spinach, Swiss chard, lettuce, watercress, endive, green beans, dandelion, cabbage, mustard greens and rocket. Various kinds of edible seaweeds are also packed with vitamins and minerals. I often add a whole dulse leaf to a casserole, brown rice, stocks, and soups. This is a great way to get extra nutritional goodness.

Eat more whole foods

These days, we all live super busy lives but to what end?

About 15 years ago, a colleague and friend made a remark that has stuck in my mind ever since. He said, 'Everyone has busy sickness. We are all involved in doing so much which prevents us from seeing clearly what we are doing and why'. After that I thought a lot about this concept of 'busy sickness' and tried to become more conscious of slowing things down in my life.

Recently, I was in the bank talking to a service manager and she asked me what work I did. I told her I was a health coach who worked with high-achieving women. She was really interested and shared with me that she wished she had more time to buy fresh whole food, but her life was so busy that it was easier to buy processed food. I realised that so many people like her are caught up in the whirl of life, trying to fit too many things in.

Many people are now aware of the importance of reviewing the amount of processed foods that may be in their diet. A more considered approach to the food you regularly consume will set you on the path to a healthy and longer life.

> *If you feel swamped with so much to do and think that you have to buy processed meals and foods to save time, here is a trick to combat this practice. Don't cut things out of your life – crowd them out step-by-step.*

It is more achievable to ease different foods out rather than by giving them up, only for you to end up reverting back to your old ways.

Whole foods are those foods that are consumed in the form that they come from nature without any processing. So what are the real benefits of reducing or removing most processed foods and replacing them with whole foods?

1. Less toxins in your body. Processed foods are full of chemicals, added sugar and preservatives that give the food flavour and a longer shelf life.

2. Food is energy for your body. You will have more energy because you are mostly eating food that has high nutritional value.

3. Food that you make from whole foods will taste better because it is fresh, and because you prepared it from scratch in your home.

4. Improved moods because most processed foods (unless specifically stated on the item) have added sugar. Sugar is well known for causing a disruption in people's blood sugar levels when too much is consumed. Sugar is not evil, but it is addictive and we are much better off when we only have small amounts.

5. Eating about 70 per cent or more whole foods will help prevent disease and slow down the aging process, because your body doesn't have to work so hard to deal with toxins or items that are not nutrients.

Here are some of my recommended easy steps for you to follow to improve your nutritional levels:

• Buy one third less processed food and replace with cooked whole foods.

• Planning and shopping for your food weekly is the key. On Sunday (or another day that suits you), check out your recipe books or find an online recipe planner for quick and easy-to-prepare healthy food, and plan all of your meals for the week. Get your partner and/or kids involved if applicable. Work on removing processed meals. At first this might only comprise 50 per cent of your processed meals, but the aim is to eventually weed most of them out.

• From your recipes, create your shopping list and then go to the supermarket (or other grocery shops), or order the food items online. There are a lot of these services available, including organic food websites.

- After you have purchased your food, cook it up in batches for the week. Again, get help from family members to chop, stir, or wash dishes. Freeze some of your prepared meals and store the rest in the fridge, ready to go.

- Eat organic produce whenever you can, or grow your own small backyard vegetable garden. It's not difficult to do. A no-dig raised garden bed about 2m x 2m is all you need to get a whole lot of fresh food growing. The nutrient value is the best it can be when you pick vegetables and eat them fresh.

- Be patient; it won't all come together at once. Have fun cooking and doing something that is going to benefit you and your family's health.

- When buying any processed foods, always check the labels so you know what you are buying. As a general rule, if the label lists more than five ingredients or you don't know what all of them are, don't buy the product.

- You don't have to cut out all processed foods, just increase your whole food intake.

Eat healthy snacks

Snacks are great and help us have sufficient energy to get through the day. Healthy snacks are even better and can be just as yummy as a piece of super sugary cake.

Here are some ideas for healthy snacks. But don't stop here – create your own:

- Fruit is the most obvious one. What fruit do you love? I love berries, especially blueberries and raspberries because they are high in anti-oxidants and fibre and low in sugar. All fruit contains sugar so aim to not exceed three pieces per day.

- Celery or carrots with hummus or tahini, peanut or almond butter are great.

- A handful of nuts. These are easy to overdo so watch the amount of nuts you eat if you are weight conscious.

- Hummus on a rice cracker or wholegrain toast if you are not following a gluten-free diet.

- Fruit and vegetable smoothies or freshly squeezed juices.

- Organic dark chocolate with 70 per cent plus cacao content.

- Olives or pickled vegetables.

- Kale or seaweed chips.

- Protein balls.

- A glass of coconut water.

Use only healthy fats

Choosing fats that are the best for your health can be confusing. The types of fats that are available are:

- saturated fats

- monounsaturated fats

- polyunsaturated fats

- trans fats.

I use cold pressed organic coconut and olive oil, grass-fed butter, ghee, and sesame oil.

Currently, there is a raging debate going on about the use of saturated fats found in animal products and coconut oil. The advantage of coconut oil is that it has a high smoking point and is good for cooking.

There are a number of research articles available to read and learn more about saturated fats. I follow the general concept that anything in moderation is ok.

The best thing to do is to check the research and make up your own mind.

Marion Nestle is Paulette Goddard Professor in the Department of Nutrition, Food Studies, and Public Health at New York University. Her article at the following website may be useful.[4]

http://www.foodpolitics.com/2014/03/
is-saturated-fat-a-problem-food-for-debate/

ABC Health and Wellbeing site has a good article on what to believe about the debate on saturated fats.[5]

http://www.abc.net.au/health/features/stories/
2013/11/04/3883432.htm

I also suggest you look into genetically modified based oils (GMOs) as there is growing concern about how they might have a disruptive effect on our health.

Overleaf is a list...

Type of fat	Benefit	Best uses
Saturated fats – coconut oil, animal products such as red meat, fish, poultry, eggs, whole milk dairy products.	Debate about whether good or harmful in large amounts. Coconut oil is considered to be very good for you as it contains lauric acids which is good for digestion and helps with weight loss.	For cooking as they are heat stable and don't oxidise at high temperatures.
Monounsatu-rated fats – olive oil, peanut oil, canola oil, safflower oil and sesame seed oil.	Good fats. Found in a variety of foods and oils. Research shows these oils benefit insulin levels, and decrease heart risk.	Raw – to add to food. I recommend staying away from any oil for cooking that is not cold pressed.
Polyunsaturated fats	Good fats. Especially Omega 3 found in cold water fish or their oil. They are extremely good for you supporting heart and brain health and reducing inflammation in the body. There are plant sources of Omega 3 in nuts, flaxseed and flaxseed oil, but it is not as available to your body as is that from fish products.	Either eat cold water fish a few times a week or (as most people do) take the supplements found in health food stores.
Trans fats or synthetic fats	No benefit. Harmful and have been removed from most processed food products such as biscuits, potato chips.	Avoid using.

Limit alcohol, sugar and coffee

We tend to love these three things. Alcohol relaxes us after a hard day at work, sugar feeds our energy, and coffee keeps us alert and awake. I have often asked myself 'Why are all the yummiest things in life somewhat problematic?' The answer I have discovered is that they are addictive and do offer short term benefits, but are not helpful in the long term if we overuse them.

The term 'in moderation' is one we often use, yet fail to obey. Indulgences like alcohol, sugar and coffee are not necessarily harmful, but when we overuse them they create problems for us. Type 2 Diabetes is a case in point.

If you feel you may be depending on any of these items in your life, you need to cross a bridge to a place where you enjoy a well-balanced diet that provides you with ample energy and vitality without relying on drugs to help you.

For example, let's say you want to give up drinking coffee but you're finding it very challenging to do; the smell, the sight of it and the urge for a 'cuppa' is just too strong, especially in social circumstances. I suggest that you try cutting back to one coffee a day and replacing the others with a good quality green tea. Green tea has caffeine in it but is full of anti-oxidants which are good for you. It is true that coffee has goodness as well; however, if you have digestive issues coffee can have a caustic effect on your gut.

After some time, you will get used to drinking green tea and then you can make that one coffee weaker or buy instant coffee and wean yourself off that way. Continue to drink green tea as an alternative until the urge to have a coffee has disappeared. I weaned myself off my craving for coffee this way so I can assure you that it works.

With alcohol, cut back by replacing it with a non-alcoholic alternative such as a Virgin Bloody Mary, Bitters, Lime and Soda or sparkling water.

With sugar, make or buy some sugar-free deserts, eat more low-sugar fruit and sweet root vegetables. These foods all have natural sugar and this will help you to wean yourself off it. Use dark organic stevia as a replacement for sugar. It makes food taste sweet and will help you to stop craving sugar.

Foods for Optimal Health

A diet that helps you to achieve the optimum state for your body includes those foods that create:

- low inflammation

- a state of alkaline pH

- correct body mass index (BMI).

If you haven't already noticed, I am passionate about preventing disease through a healthy diet and informed lifestyle choices. I feel this way because many chronic illnesses (otherwise known as lifestyle illnesses) are preventable. What you eat and drink plays a huge role in preventing disease or causing it. Knowing this drives me to help high-achieving women to make critical lifestyle and dietary shifts so they can live a full and productive life.

One of the key cornerstones of optimum health is to ensure your body has very low levels of inflammation. Dr Andrew Weil, MD is a strong advocate of eating healthy foods to reduce chronic inflammation. He highlights the association between chronic inflammation and many illnesses, including heart disease, Alzheimer's, and many forms of cancer. He also explains in clear terms that chronic inflammation is not what occurs in the body as localised swelling, redness, and pain. This form of inflammation has an important purpose in healing the body from injury or infection. In contrast, chronic inflammation is silent and is principally caused by stress, lack of exercise, smoking and toxic chemicals in the environment.

Dr Weil also says that what we eat plays a big role in either preventing inflammation or promoting it. Dr Weil's website: www.drweil.com is a great resource for all things about nutrition.[6]

Although many health coaches, health practitioners, and physicians are doing all they can to help people to change their diets and their lifestyles, we still seem to be going backwards. Current statistics from the Centre for Disease Control and Prevention in the USA indicate that 86 per cent of their health care dollars are spent treating chronic health conditions. In 2009, the Australian Institute for Health and Welfare published statistics showing that Australia spent 120 billion dollars on health that year compared to 600 million dollars in 1999.[7]

In my opinion, the writing is on the wall. Unless we take this situation into our own hands, things are not going to turn around and improve. And we are all paying the price for unhealthy lifestyle choices through our taxes and through our own diseases. Yet, we have become so used to stress, poor sleep, not-so-great diets, and up and down exercise. I also know that depression and anxiety play a role in inflammation in the body as well.

In this chapter, my focus has been to demonstrate to you how you can change the food you eat to reduce inflammation and help your body to stay disease-free and healthy.

Foods to eat	Foods to reduce
Eat a wide variety of fruits and vegetables on a daily basis.	Minimise processed and junk foods as much you can. Start small and keep going.
Eat whole grains, beans and legumes and pasta.	Processed grains in many forms such as cereals, white breads.
Consume healthy fats and oils daily in small amounts.	Minimise fried foods, cakes, sweet biscuits and any processed foods.

Lean protein from fish, poultry, and beef.	
Drink pure water, or drinks that are mostly water.	Limit coffee, alcohol and sugar.
If you are vegan or vegetarian, substitute protein-rich vegetables and soy products for meat, and use a high-quality vegan protein powder.	

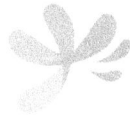

Chapter 6
Deciphering Cravings and Addictions

As a general principle, craving something is not bad. Cravings occur for a wide range of reasons; however, they always exist to inform us about our body and our life.

The purpose of this book is to help you understand that your body is your expert; your job is to tune into it, along with your mind and spirit. If you do, you will no longer have an ongoing struggle with weight gain or mood swings. You will want to look after all of you. You will thrive and develop a strong immune system, a healthy gut, and a life filled with possibilities – no matter how young or old you are.

Right now, you might be starting out on your health journey or getting back on track. You need to remember that cravings are part of life. It is how we relate to them and the actions we take as a result of them that matter.

Understanding Cravings

The initial step is to understand your current cravings. Take a look at your diet – what foods do you crave? What is missing in your life?

What are you craving because of the deficits in your life? And what are your behaviors? What actions do you take when you crave something? Do you unconsciously eat it, do it, or act on it?

Here are some suggestions to help you to better understand what are causing your cravings:

1. **Water:** If you are not drinking enough water, you become dehydrated. Dehydration can cause a feeling of mild hunger; a craving for something. Instead of eating try drinking a big glass of water first. The opposite is also true; excess water can also cause cravings. The trick is to create a balanced water intake.

2. **Low nutrients:** If your body is missing certain nutrients, it will crave them, so this is something you should be aware of. A lot of people crave salt. Sometimes this involves a certain vegetable. Other common cravings are sugar, chocolate and coffee. While these foods are addictive, the perceived need for them is often due to an overall imbalance in nutritional levels. When we have a diversity of nutrients in our diet, cravings of all kinds are not usually present.

3. **Seasonal:** Cravings are associated with the seasons which, in turn, are part of a varied life. Getting in tune with the seasons and your diet is marvelous. I have a few seasonal cookbooks and I love them. We often crave foods that balance the elements of each season. Naturally, in summer people crave cooling foods like fruit, raw food, and refreshing drinks. In autumn, people crave grounding foods like onions, nuts, and squash. In winter, we crave warming foods like stews, fats and oils, while in spring, we crave detoxifying foods like leafy greens.

4. **Lifestyle:** This is an area we often pay lip service to, but it can have a huge impact on our health. If we are not happy in a relationship, bored, feeling stressed, uninspired in our work, listless, engaging in exercise that doesn't suit us, disconnected, or low in our Spirit, we may attempt to fill the gap with cravings

for food. This is called emotional eating, and many people are familiar with it. We do it to fill the 'hole' in our life. It takes courage and fortitude to deal with the real reasons for the 'holes' in our life. To act is to face the unknown and that is often scary.

5. **Hormonal:** Cravings are common for women when they are menstruating, pregnant, or during menopause. This is due to fluctuating testosterone and estrogen levels which can cause unique and unusual cravings.

6. **Foods that remind us of our past:** When we eat foods reminiscent of our childhood, we often develop a craving for them. You can experiment with these foods and develop a modern, healthy way of preparing then. Foods from earlier times when there was little or no processing involved are currently undergoing a revival.

7. **Yin-Yang imbalance:** Yin foods tend to be cooling and moistening, whereas Yang foods are warming and dryer. If we eat too many of one type of food, an imbalance is created causing us to crave the opposite type of food. For example, eating too many raw foods (Yin) can cause cravings for over-cooked foods that are dehydrating (Yang) and vice versa.

When you get more in touch with your cravings, you are connecting on a much deeper level with your body. Everyone experiences cravings: sometimes this is for addictive foods and substances in our life which can occur because we are out of balance in our foods, in our emotions, and in our life.

Cravings are like a messenger; they tell us something about what our body needs more or less of. Enjoy connecting with your cravings and your body. As a result, you will finally be able to unravel the mystery of their source.

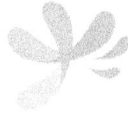

Chapter 7
Simple Tactics to Lose Weight without Dieting

Losing weight and keeping it off is one of the big problems that many people face in their lives today. I belong to the camp that says it is better to strive for a healthy, vibrant body, than to focus singularly on losing weight.

For 20 years of my life, I was locked into a 'weight on, weight off' circular pattern of dieting and unable to keep excess weight off. My weight never varied by more than 10 kilos, but it always went up and down. These days, I have now settled at my correct weight and reset my body to stay that way. The key for me was to remove sugar from my diet.

Previously, my habit was to eat sugar, put on weight, diet, lose weight, and then return to eating sugar. I knew sugar was problematic but I was addicted to it. As we now know, sugar and simple carbohydrates have a major impact on our blood sugar levels which, in turn, affect our weight, moods, sleep, and general wellbeing. I still consume a small amount of sugar but nothing like the levels I unconsciously ate previously. In fact, my palette has changed and I can only tolerate a small amount of sweet foods such as is in 90 per cent cacao dark chocolate. I absolutely love dark chocolate and can eat it without guilt, knowing that my body likes it also.

You may now be realising that when we crowd certain substances out of our daily diet, over time our palette does change to enjoy the new healthy foods and dislike what we loved previously. This is how I did it in my own life with the substances that were not nourishing me – sugar, coffee, gluten, and dairy. I no longer have addictions, cravings, and feelings of missing out on the yummy things in life. Instead, I have new and improved good things I enjoy. I love healthy snacks and as far as my comfort foods are concerned, I have just adopted the healthy versions.

Life is not about giving things up. This is unrealistic and only leaves you feeling defeated and stuck. Instead, crowd out what doesn't nourish your life – substances, things, habits, people, mindsets, and anything else you want to systematically shed over time. Do this and you can expect to feel more powerful, more vital, and more in control of your life.

It is only since I started on my journey into discovering what helps my body to thrive that I have achieved my normal body weight without any major fluctuations. I no longer have rollercoaster weight problems, or blood sugar highs and lows. I live my life with ease and I feel much happier and love myself more. Partly this is the result of feeling and looking better; however, mostly I have healed myself from disliking my body, and feeling fat and uncomfortable. I have a much greater connection and love for my body now.

My Personal Journey to Improve My Health and Wellbeing

So how did I transform my own health and my life? I decided to kick-start this process of adjusting my eating patterns by doing something that was challenging but that felt right for me. I went on a ten-day juice fast consisting mostly of vegetables, with a small amount of low sugar fruit added. I followed Joe Cross's guidelines[8] and, admittedly, the first two days were difficult while toxins from coffee and sugar left my body. In 2012, I lost eight kilos in ten days and I have never regained it. I managed to reset my body to the correct weight for me. I lost my cravings for sugar and never resumed eating bread, cakes, biscuits, and other processed simple carbohydrates. I made the decision to change a few things in my diet and it worked well for me. As a result, I have never been happier or felt as healthy.

> *We are all unique beings because of our genetics and environment – and so there is no one diet that fits all.*

The secret to thriving from nutrition is to experiment with different types of healthy foods and observe those that make you feel good, energise you, and your body seems to love. This process can be developed and refined over time. Just having the intent to do this, will lead you to increase your understanding of what nourishes your body.

There are of course guidelines for optimum health, but within that range we can find and choose the foods that our bodies best thrive on. This is true for losing weight as well. A body that is being given highly nutritional food will lose weight over time as needed.

Weight loss is usually a by-product of taking small steps to modify our health. I know many women have tried all sorts of different diets and other weight loss regimes and aren't able to shift excess weight.

It is a complex problem with many contributing factors playing a role, including emotional, mental and physiological issues. Becoming healthier and leaner is an option available for everyone in their lives, and is a goal you can work towards.

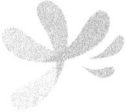

NOURISH YOUR BODY FOR YOUR IDEAL SIZE – JENNY'S STORY

Jenny is an amazing high-achieving woman. She has lived a relatively charmed life with things always falling into place for her. She has always remained positive about life and her relationships with people and, as a result, things almost always have gone her way. She is a great contributor to the community and is a very successful business owner. In her work life, she mostly dealt with men and didn't really worry too much about fussing over her appearance. Jenny has been fortunate to be able to dictate the terms of her life – mostly.

Jenny came to see me after making a decision that it was time to do something about her health. She was experiencing problems with:

- low energy and feeling a bit negative
- sluggish and carrying too much weight
- no regular exercise
- feeling flat and lacking in confidence.

The first thing Jenny wanted to work on with me was her energy levels. She was aware that everything in life depends on having enough energy, and if she wanted to be highly productive in life, she needed to address that.

While working on her health concerns together, the goal was to initially fix her immediate problems and for Jenny to move to the next level of productivity, creativity and life in general.

Jenny started to keep a record of all of her meals and snacks, and how her energy and mood felt after eating. This exercise revealed to her that there was a correlation between low energy and eating wheat or products that have wheat in them. As a result of this finding, Jenny cut out gluten from her diet. The outcome was that she had greatly improved energy levels and felt more positive about her life.

At the same time, Jenny started exercising for half an hour three days a week. Not being someone who enjoys exercise for the sake of it, she needed to do something she really loved. She loved riding her bike so it became a fun thing to do every day. After about two weeks she felt fantastic and her clothes were starting to feel loose.

Keeping the steps simple and not overloading herself, Jenny finally felt motivated to tackle her weight issue with persistence. We both recognised that her weight was not shifting easily, even though her body was slimming down. So we decided to remove all grains and sugars from her diet, upped the amount of exercise she was doing to five days a week and lowered her alcohol intake.

At this point, things started to feel a bit restrictive when she went out for a meal and the adjustment was slow. Jenny felt that it was better for her to tackle her weight in a slow and deliberate way, and that ultimately it was not about how much she lost and how quickly. Rather, she adopted the mindset that she was on a journey to change her eating and lifestyle patterns to support a healthy, active and more productive life. She recognised that dieting was pointless and that she had to develop a good understanding about what her body needed to maintain her optimum health.

Consequently, we added in some goals around loving and nurturing her body every day to change her attitude towards herself. She began to love her body and not to feel 'lumpy' in it. She recognized how beautiful she really was, and, as a result, her self-care started to feel more natural. As people increasingly commented on how fantastic she looked, she developed a new-found interest in her appearance and grooming.

Jenny learnt how to nourish her body and how to keep her weight down to a level where she felt energised and happy. These days, her whole eating regime has changed and has become the normal way for her to live. Since modifying her eating patterns, she has gone on to do more than she'd originally intended, and she has felt renewed with a new vitality and purpose. Life is full of possibilities for Jenny once again.

Simple Tips to Lose Weight Without Dieting

Drink more water

Dehydration and hunger are often confused. Whether severe or mild, dehydration does affect your body's metabolism. You should aim to drink eight glasses of water each day. It's also good to drink most in the morning, less in the afternoon, and less in the evening so that you don't lose sleep going to the toilet all night. In addition, it is advisable to minimise other drinks such as coffee and soft drinks. To help deal with hunger, drink water instead of eating something and see if this takes away the hunger. Also, drink water before meals. This will also help to stop you overeating.

Eat breakfast

Eating a good healthy breakfast is one of the best things you can do to set you up properly for your day. If we miss breakfast, we are usually hungry by mid-morning and we reach for unhealthy snacks.

A nutritious and filling breakfast is one that includes some protein, complex carbohydrates and healthy fats. If life is too busy in the morning, a healthy smoothie is always a good option. The important thing is to make sure you have something at breakfast. If you are not a breakfast person, preferring to consume a coffee on the run, it is time to crowd that habit out at a pace that works for you.

Eat real carbohydrates

This is a great health tip and works well for most people. Replace refined carbohydrates from white products like bread, pasta, cereal, cakes, biscuits, chips, with complex carbohydrates including vegetables, fruits, whole grains, nuts, seeds, and legumes. These foods slow down digestion and this helps to stablise blood sugar levels in your body. Vegetables and fruits are high in fibre which also aids digestion, and are packed with anti-oxidants which reduce invisible inflammation in the body. These are all whole foods.

Choose healthy fats

It is now well recognised that healthy fats are good for you and that we actually need fats in our diet for energy, vitamin absorption, healthy hair, skin and nails, and normal bodily functions. Good fats include extra virgin olive oil, virgin coconut oil, ghee, nuts, seeds, fish, and avocado. These fats help to lower blood pressure, reduce cholesterol levels, and protect us from heart disease, cancer, depression and Alzheimer's disease.

Eat healthy protein

Proteins, in the form of amino acids, are the building blocks for life. Our bodies are made of protein and we need it to power our energy and renew the cells in our body. For omnivores, the richest forms of protein are found in animal products including meat, dairy, eggs, and fish. It is also found in beans, nuts and seeds. From a health perspective, it is best to eat meat that has been pasture-raised, free range, or organic if you can afford it. For vegetarians, the food choices for protein include eggs and yoghurt. For vegans and vegetarians, tofu, tempeh, and peanut butter are good sources of protein, along with nuts, seeds and legumes.

Get plenty of sleep

Lack of sleep disrupts circadian rhythms and can lead to inefficient body regulation of energy balance, metabolism and appetite. Many of our bodily functions are unsettled when we don't sleep well. Work out how many hours of sleep you need to operate at your peak and do your best to get that amount. Seven to eight hours of sleep each night is a good amount for most people.

Cook more regularly

Cooking can be very relaxing and creative, and cooking more regularly at home is really important to help with weight loss. This way you have control over ingredients and portion sizes. I recommend making a food plan for recipes each week; shop for ingredients and cook in batches to freeze or store meals for the week in the fridge. In addition, plan for one evening out during the week where you choose healthy foods. If you are too busy to cook all the time, take this process step-by-step, first by making a start to cook more frequently and shop for recipes. Experimenting with different foods is also a way to get more satisfaction and enjoyment out of cooking.

Exercise your body and mind

Of course, you need to move your body and create a positive mindset for your life if you are to lose weight and keep it off. Find the type of movement that turns you on. Walking, yoga, swimming, and working with a personal trainer are all good. So is choosing to walk more as part of your daily routine: walk to the shops for extra things, take the stairs instead of lifts, and keep your body moving through the day as much as you can. Instead of watching television, read something inspirational. You might also like to try meditation or go for walks in nature.

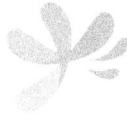

Chapter 8
Sleep Well by Tweaking your Nutrition

Sleep is so important to your general wellbeing that without it, pretty much everything else in your life falls apart. Yet, in today's frenetic world, we try to manage on less and less sleep as we attempt to get more and more done. Somewhere, we seem to have wrongly deduced that sleep is not all that important.

A few years ago, I felt as though my brain was on alert for 24 hours a day. I was wired during the day and, during my sleep, I was thinking and sleeping at the same time. I guess I probably averaged about three hours of actual sleep every night. This went on for weeks. I never felt rested. I couldn't think properly, couldn't remember things very well, and ended up with adrenal fatigue, which persisted for quite some time.

Finally, I woke up to the problem and sought help. And, as it turned out, the answer I discovered was surprising. I was an extreme case but, generally speaking, I find that high-achieving women often try to cut corners with their sleep by frequently working late at night. Yet, getting a good night's sleep is not an option; it is an essential factor which enables your body to function normally.

Sleep Needs Fuel

To most of us, sleep seems like a passive process. We don't often realise that it requires energy to do its job. While we are passively asleep, a very active process is underway in our body.

There are at least two very important functions that sleep performs:

- It repairs cells and restores the body in readiness to be able to function properly the next day.
- It enables the brain to process information, lay down memory, and enable learning.

Without proper sleep, we become stressed and have difficulty functioning properly at work and in our daily lives.

The inability to sleep properly is often due to stress, an over-active mind, and certain bad habits like working late at night. Many people resort to sleeping tablets, Melatonin, and other supplements in an attempt to be able to sleep well at night. Personally, I've tried Melatonin but I found that it made me feel very tired the next day. So when I discovered a nutritional way of dealing with the problem I was amazed and very happy that it didn't involve popping a pill.

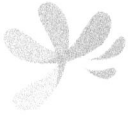

THE IMPORTANCE OF SLEEP FOR OPTIMAL PERFORMANCE – VANESSA'S STORY

Vanessa was a high-flying corporate executive with a large bank, heading up the Corporate Social Responsibility Program. She loved her job which involved working with a team, making a difference in people's lives, and plenty of travel to meet leaders of exciting sustainably projects as prospective partners with the bank.

After about eight months into the role, life for Vanessa became even busier to the point where she had to work back late in the office more than the occasional few hours. She was still engrossed in her work and didn't really notice the extra workload, but eventually the daily hours became 10–12 hours and she also started working weekends.

Returning home from work most nights after 8.00 pm meant that Vanessa often didn't have enough time or energy to cook dinner. Instead, she would fill her freezer with prepared meals from the supermarket that simply required her to heat and eat them. Sometimes, she would just have muesli for dinner while she was busy reading one of her team member's reports.

As opportunities for social engagements and exercise diminished, and as the computer screen increasingly dominated her life, Vanessa's health started to deteriorate. The quality of her sleep started to suffer: she found herself waking up thinking about all the things she hadn't finished at work, and then she couldn't easily get back to sleep. She started to feel more stressed, and really tired and empty the next morning. She couldn't remember the last time she had been for a run or to the gym, and she avoided getting on the scales to see the effects of no exercise. Contact with friends became via text messages. To compensate, she would tell herself that things would return to normal soon.

Vanessa still felt that the work issue was a temporary thing so she kept giving it all. However, the situation didn't improve and in fact things actually got busier at work. She lost team members and then as a result of being understaffed, she was required to take on extra work to meet her supervisors' expectations. Gradually, due to her poor sleep and diet, as well as lack of exercise, Vanessa's work productivity began to suffer. At this point, Vanessa still wasn't aware of what was happening in her life; she was still totally immersed in what she had to do, rather than what was going on. She was caught up in a world she couldn't really see a clear way out of. Her perspective had narrowed so she felt she was in a deep valley with cliffs all around her: she couldn't climb out or get high enough to see the view.

Vanessa eventually hit the wall. She was wired and tired all the time, short-tempered with her work team, sleep deprived, not eating well and having a few drinks every night to help her relax. Her body was becoming exhausted: her adrenal glands were not keeping up with the constant stress, her memory was slipping and she started to resent her work. She often felt numb to everything and would sit and stare at the wall in the evenings.

Finally, after more than a year feeling like this, she experienced an incident at work with her boss, which shocked her into going to the doctor. He immediately identified that Vanessa was suffering from high blood pressure, chronic exhaustion, depression, and anxiety. He advised her to take three weeks off work to rest, sleep and reconsider her life, and he suggested she think seriously about her work/life balance. He also told her this short break would help to restore her temporarily; however, she needed to carefully review her whole life and change a number of things about it. He recommended she have counselling and consider her job options.

How Can You Restore Good Sleep Patterns?

If you are in a situation like Vanessa's, sleep is the first thing you need to attend to. The first step is give your body the right fuel at the right times. This will restore your energy for sleep and over a few weeks, re-train your body to sleep normally again.

Once your sleep patterns are well-established, you will feel so much better. However, problems will return if you don't review your lifestyle and change any problem areas that were the initial cause of your sleep problems.

My 10 Top Tips for Restoring Sleep the Safe and Simple Way

The following advice is for people who are generally in good health but suffer from stress, overthinking, and habits which don't support sleep. It is *not* recommended for people who have clinical health conditions like sleep apnea, depression or any other serious health issues. Always consult your doctor if you have serious health problems.

Depending on the severity of your sleep problems, follow this advice for three to five weeks. Remember the aim of this method is to help you rebuild enough energy to get your body back into the sleep 'black'.

1. Eat three meals a day as you normally would.

2. If you exercise before breakfast, always have something small to eat beforehand – maybe half a piece of fruit or a protein ball. If you neglect to do this, you can be setting yourself up for an energy deficit. Your sleep 'budget' starts with fueling your body from the start of the day. If you exercise in the early morning without having some fuel from food, your body remains in a catch-up mode throughout the day.

3. In between meals have fruit juice without added sugar on hand

to sip (approximately one glass per day). This practice will provide your body with readily available energy at frequent intervals. You won't need to do this for the rest of your life; the idea is that you do this for a specific amount of time – just until you are sleeping properly again.

4. Before bed have a small supper. **This is a must.** You could have a glass of warm milk, with or without cocao, stewed fruit, a coconut ball, or a couple of fresh dates. **NOTE:** If you have sensitivity to dairy or gluten, ensure that you are not accidently eating food that contain these items.

5. If you wake up in the night – get up and have a snack such as a date, a protein ball, a glass of milk or other small item – not junk or processed food. Minimise your alertness by going quietly and quickly to get something to eat and then return to bed. This will help you get back to sleep straight away.

Good sleep habits

6. Wind down in the evening. No work on devices or over-stimulation of your brain. Do any of the following: meditation, deep breathing, listening to soothing music, or watching something on television that makes you laugh.

7. Go to bed no later than 10.00 pm and to sleep no later than 10.30pm.

8. Do not keep active devices in your bedroom, especially near your head.

9. Make sure your room is dark and that your bed is comfortable.

10. To help with locating the source of your active mind, you could try keeping a journal of your thoughts throughout the day for a

couple of days. It takes effort to become aware of your thoughts; you will be rewarded with clarity and understanding about what you are thinking, and how much you push your brain. Doing this will help you to understand what is driving your overactive mind.

My suggestion is that you follow this sleep restoration program for three to five weeks, depending on your individual results. You will need to commit to this program and do it properly as your body needs this energy. Once your sleep patterns have returned to normal, make sure that you continue to keep up these good sleep habits. Remember, sleep is the number one activity for enabling you to function properly throughout your day.

Diagnose the Initial Cause of your Sleep Problems

The method I have outlined above is the 'how to' for restoring your sleep and is a good starting point to get you back to normal sleep patterns. However, you also need to uncover why you have developed poor sleep. In this way, you will be able to work on modifying your lifestyle and making sure that you change any unhealthy habits for good.

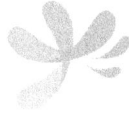

Chapter 9
The Gut Health Revolution

Whoever you are and no matter how well you may currently feel, now is the right time to set about improving your digestive health. If you have ever had antibiotics, a serious virus, become sensitive to gluten, dairy or other foods, or just feel plain tired and worn out, it is likely that you have something going on in your gut. Digestive issues are rife in most of the population, and the spectrum of issues is wide ranging, from mild to severe and chronic.

Despite this there is good news. There have been some remarkable insights occurring recently in the field of digestive health research and practice.

What is the Human Microbiome?

The human microbiome is the collection of trillions of microbes that live within us and on us. According to Dr Jason Hawrelak (a naturopath, western herbalist, researcher and educator), the microbiota living in our gut are the farmers and guards that protect us from pathogens.[9]

It is only very recently that scientists have started to map the human microbiome and understand its function. It's actually a genetic revolution, as scientists establish the exact composition and genetic content of our microbiome using advanced technology that is cheaper and quicker than when they previously sequenced the human genome.

Our microbiome has trillions of microbiota comprised of a variety of different strains. Our digestive systems contain good and bad bacteria, as well as neutral bacteria. All of them are important to maintain our health, but problems occur when the good ones are compromised. When we take antibiotics or other medications, become chronically stressed, or get a nasty virus, we weaken our microbiota. We change its composition and, as a result, the gut 'farmers' and 'protectors' drop in numbers and the pathogens start to dominate. This is where problems with our digestive health can start to occur.

Our Microbiome – the Key to Preventing Illness

There is so much more information available now about the value of our microbiome: what it is and what happens to it when we neglect it, and how to rebuild it to boost our overall health. With our current knowledge, you and I can be aware of any changes in our health in relation to changes in our gut health. In many cases, what is occurring in your gut may be the source of problems elsewhere in your body. Our brain and other important parts of our body are reliant on our microbiome protecting us. Conversely, they are vulnerable once our gut is compromised.

In my work as an integrative nutrition health coach, I see many women who suffer from thyroid diseases. Plus, I have personally experienced Hashimoto's Thyroiditis, (an autoimmune disease) since 2009. Initially, I wasn't able to find any way of improving or reversing this debilitating disease. I was advised by doctors and other health professionals that there was no cure for it.

In early 2015, I participated in a new health program in the USA which centered on healing the gut and reestablishing the intestinal microbiome. After six weeks, I'd completed the program and had my thyroid tested again. To my great surprise (and to my doctors), the tests revealed that my thyroid, and the antibodies associated with it, had recovered substantially during that period. At that moment, I received the best news of my life: I had concrete evidence of the relationship between gut health and autoimmune disease. My doctor said to me: 'Whatever you are doing, keep doing it!' I am now working on the 'finishing touches' to fully reverse Hashimoto's Thyroiditis disease and come off medication completely.

In many health practitioner circles, it is now an accepted fact that many (if not all) diseases have their origins in the gut. Over the last two decades, research has demonstrated that gut health is critical to overall health and wellness, and that an unhealthy gut contributes to a wide range of diseases including diabetes, obesity, many autoimmune diseases, depression, chronic fatigue and more.

Building a healthy digestive system is one of the most important things you can do to protect yourself from pathogens, toxins, viruses, diseases and any imbalances that living in the 21st Century places on your body. If you decide to make your gut health a high priority, you will be on the path to ensuring that you are protected from many diseases.

Before I discuss the cause of gut problems, it is important to dig a bit deeper to understand two important aspects of digestive health: the microbial activity of your gut and the mucosa or gut barrier.

The microbial activity of your gut

Functional nutritionist, Andrea Nakayama has described four kinds of microbial activities that go on amongst the trillions of microbes that live in your gut and act to either keep it healthy or unhealthy:

- **Mutualism:** This is where the microbes and our bodies are mutually benefiting each other. For example, when we eat fermented vegetables that contain these microbes, both parties benefit. The mutualistic organisms get nourishment, and they then produce nutrients that benefit our bodies.

- **Commensalism:** In a commensal relationship, one organism in the relationship benefits, and the other one is neither benefitted nor harmed – it is neutral.

- **Parasitism:** A parasitic relationship is where one organism benefits at the expense of another (the host). The impact of parasitism on us as the host can vary from minor to severe.

- **Pathogenic:** A pathogenic relationship is where an organism causes damage to our body through infection. If your body is already impaired, an opportunistic pathogen will cause disease. In a healthy body, the pathogen is rendered harmless; however, it can take advantage when our defenses are down. This mostly occurs when the beneficial microbes are destroyed by antibiotics, or when the immune system has been suppressed by drug treatment or other illnesses.

The mucosa or the gut barrier

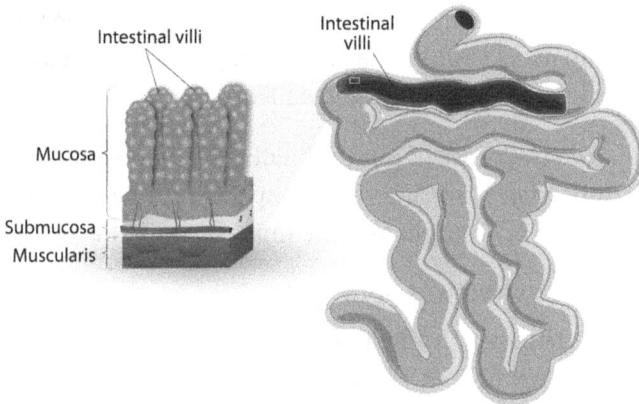

Your digestive tract is a tube that extends through your body and is totally separate from it. Everything you eat and drink flows through this tube for the purpose of digesting what you consume and allowing all the microscopic nutrients to be absorbed into your body. The tube wall is built of an amazing lining called the mucosa which protects your body from substances moving through the wall into the blood stream and into your body.

The good bacteria are like soldiers that guard and protect the mucosa from anything getting through to your body. In a healthy system this works well. However, in an unhealthy gut, toxins can force their way through the mucosal wall and enter into the bloodstream. The term for this is 'leaky gut'. Once this happens, allergies, arthritis and a whole range of other illnesses become a real threat. This is a very common scenario and most people aren't even aware it is happening.

Seven clues that your digestive system may not be functioning well

1.   You have taken antibiotics recently, or on occasions throughout your life.

2.   You feel tired or bloated after eating.

3.   You have been feeling stressed for some time.

4.   Your diet is high in processed foods.

5.   You already have an autoimmune disease, or are consulting your doctor to investigate this possibility.

6.   You have an irritable bowel that fluctuates between constipation and diarrhea.

7.   Your energy is low and you don't know why.

Common mistakes that cause people to ignore important signals from their bodies

They:

- feel low in energy and just think it is part of life, getting older, or just a bad patch that will eventually go away

- don't know much about digestive health, and they have seen the ads on TV that suggest all you need to do is take a few probiotics to clear up gas or tummy problems

- think this 'digestive health thing' is another diet fad thing and seems a bit far-fetched

- are frightened that something terrible is wrong with them, and they really don't want to face what it might be

- have brain fog (which is very common with gut-related issues) and cannot think clearly about what steps to take regarding their health

- are out of touch with their bodies, stressed, overworking and have no time to think about their health

- don't care about their health. What is most important to them is living the 'good life' and working hard.

All of these mistakes are common to many of us. I was someone who previously didn't consider my health to be a priority and was a chronic workaholic. What's more, I'd had two warnings before I took action. It wasn't until a doctor and a naturopath both told me I was heading for a 'train wreck' that I resolved to improve my health.

When I finally acted, I had crossed many thresholds in my body, including being diagnosed with an autoimmune disease, experiencing depression, adrenal fatigue, and poor sleep. I felt stupid, ashamed, and angry with myself for being so negligent, and then had to deal with these emotions as well. In my darkest moments I remember thinking: 'If only someone had told me about all of this health stuff.'

I now feel that I have come through the looking glass to healing my body, mind and spirit. It is a never-ending journey and I have gained so much by the experience. This is why I am so passionate about helping women to avoid the health and life crisis that I experienced.

Don't wait until something bad happens to your health. Act now to improve it and it will pay off in the long-term through your quality of life and wellbeing.

Solutions

The number of people suffering from gut issues is on the rise. It is part and parcel of living in a toxic world. Many people don't even know that they have a problem, yet the tell-tale signs are there. My wish for all of my clients (and people in general) is that they will better understand the importance of gut health and decide to value and build a relationship with their intestinal microbiome. This is the path to stable and vital health to keep you in top-notch condition so you can lead a long and productive life.

These days, gut health is becoming quite trendy and there are lots of fermented foods on the market, as well as probiotics and bone broths. The important thing to note is that taking probiotics and fermented foods at the start of a gut healing process won't help greatly, especially if you have a toxic gut with high levels of candida and other pathogens.

Tips for Healing Your Gut:

1. If you suspect you may have a problem with your gut after reading the seven clues, you need to make time to get things checked out.

2. Consider having a full panel of tests done to test for candida, worms and parasites (stool test), thyroid, adrenal glands and cortisol levels, liver, kidney and heart health, vitamin D and

B's, and other tests that your doctor can advise you about. Tests are an excellent place to start to review your health status and Medicare will cover many of them.

3. If something shows up in the tests, see your doctor. If your test comes up positive for candida, bacteria, worms or parasites, there are alternatives to antibiotics. Consult a health practitioner that works with digestive health. You can still follow the guidelines outlined in this book as they are part of a digestive health protocol that will help you to improve your overall wellbeing. Working with both your doctor and a health practitioner is a good practice to ensure you get the best possible support.

4. Keep a food/mood journal for five days to check for gluten and dairy sensitivity. There are other food sensitivities; however, these two are the most common. If you eat wheat or dairy products and feel low in energy after eating them, your journal will indicate that there is a direct relationship.

5. Run an experiment, by giving up gluten and/or dairy for a couple of weeks. This is sufficient time for your energy and vitally levels to return. If they do, then it is up to you to make choices to exclude or greatly reduce these items from you diet. In many cases, once your gut is healed, you can resume eating them, but often it is best to at least eliminate gluten from your diet.

6. Consider doing a chicken or beef bone broth fast for 2–4 days. If you Google bone broths you will find plenty of recipes. You can eat steamed veggies during this period also. Google the value of bone broth. It is remarkable for the body in many ways. You can make the broth yourself. It takes some work but it is worth it. Alternatively, you can buy 100 per cent organic bone broth from the Broth for Life website (www.brothforlife.com.au).[10]

7. Eat mostly whole foods (foods that nature produces without any additives). Ensure your diet is 50 per cent vegetables (especially

green ones), 25 per cent protein, and 25 per cent complex carbohydrates such as brown rice and quinoa. Try to remove simple carbohydrates (white processed ones) from your diet.

8. Cook with unrefined coconut oil and use extra virgin olive oil on your salads.

9. Reduce sugar to not more than 5 teaspoons a day. Better still, purchase some Stevia drops and use this instead.

10. Limit your fruit intake to low-fructose fruits such as berries, kiwi fruit and green apples, and have no more than 2–3 pieces a day.

11. Drink plenty of water. Cut down on coffee and alcohol. Drink a glass of pure coconut water each day that is free from any added sugar or preservatives.

12. Exercise for at least 30 minutes for 3–5 days per week. Walking is excellent for your health.

13. Get plenty of rest and sleep. Relax more, and consider meditation and yoga.

14. Depending on what your blood and other tests reveal you should get re-tested once you have improved your diet with the right healing supplements for a certain period.

All of this information might seem overwhelming to you right now. That's ok. The knowledge is there for you to read through and consider in your own time.

I know it is more fun to check out the latest smoothie recipe or the newest trend in healthy eating. However, none of these options are going to repair your gut if you have pathogens present in your gut and are not very well. Taking action with medical doctors and a good trusted health practitioner will help you to get back on top of your health and your life – hopefully for good.

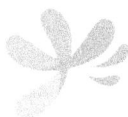

Chapter 10
Move your Body to Get Fit

Unless your job or business directly involves exercise as part of your daily routine, you are likely to be spending long hours sitting in front of a computer, doing, thinking, talking, and writing, which places a fair bit of stress on the body. Have you noticed how many chiropractors and osteopaths there are in your local area these days? It's because our computer-based lifestyles and work lives often lead to back problems, poor posture, chronic aches and pains, muscle tightness and constipation.

I'm sure we are all aware of the benefits of exercise in our life; yet somehow it often drops down on our list of priorities, particularly if we travel a lot for work, work late in the evenings, and generally feel too tired to exercise.

Here are a few reminders of just how beneficial moving your body regularly is, and the different ways that you can incorporate exercise into your life.

Exercise and movement:

- releases built up physical tension
- restores regular bowel movements
- helps with weight loss and body tone
- improves energy
- prevents heart disease and lifestyle diseases such as Type 2 diabetes
- improves mood and overall wellbeing.

The key is to develop an exercise program that fits with your body type and is something you really enjoy doing. Swimming, walking, dancing, yoga and daily stretching are great activities. If you are out of your routine due to travel or some other call on your time, you can always increase the amount of time you exercise in your room, or spend time walking. From a hotel in any city around the world you can make a point of walking everywhere, and you can increase every opportunity to use the stairs.

As your exercise or movement journey continues, it is important to increase your awareness of those activities that your body thrives on.

You will develop your knowledge of what your body thrives on by doing what you enjoy most, feel good about and want to do, again and again.

Research shows that regular movement and moderate exercise promote a healthy lifestyle and lead to improvements in wellbeing. For this reason, you might like to set some life goals for yourself such as: 'I always take the stairs instead lifts or escalators'. It's so interesting to see how few people do this at train stations or airports. I have watched and my estimate is that only around 10 – 15 per cent of people bother to do this. This is a simple yet powerful form of exercise you can easily do, which I believe sets you up for good habits and reminds you to stay active. In contrast, taking the lift or using the car when you could walk, promotes a more sedentary life. My goal of always taking the stairs has become my reminder to always try to live a more active life.

There are some wonderful case studies about longevity that occur in the Blue Zones – examples of ways of life and places around the world where people live healthy lives up to and beyond 100 years of age. My favourite example is from Sardinia where one of the things that has contributed to people living very long lifespans is their commitment to physically challenge themselves with movement. Apart from keeping generally active, they continue to take long and steep stone stairways that lead to their homes everyday. I recommend that you investigate www.bluezones.com. The case studies are rich in knowledge and very heart warming.

I love the Blue Zone case studies because they demonstrate real-world examples of how health and longevity is a natural and integrative way of life (combining both nutrition and lifestyle) versus a life that is about constantly striving for optimum health. The Blue Zone examples are like a great mystery – the quiet and unremarkable approach, yet very obvious when we enquire more deeply into how people from these areas live long hearty lives.

Think about removing complications that keep you from truly being yourself and opting for the simple, heartfelt and joyous aspects of your life.

My philosophy is to follow the Five Principles of Integrative Health I have outlined in this book as a way of finding your own personal 'Blue

Zone'. This approach incorporates a natural way of being healthy and vital for your whole life time, where you live in accordance with your unique self, and where you feel at home with your body and your life.

In this chapter, I have recommended some simple ways to get in touch with the form of exercise that best suits your body.

1. **Think about the kind of exercise you enjoyed as a child.** This is a good place to start when you are pondering what best suits you. What did you find fun and what seemed easy for you to do?

2. **Listen to your body.** Just like food, there are different forms of movement that best suit our body type. With this in mind, try to find what exercise activity works well for you. Some people need high energy, intense exercise like triathlons and long distance running. Other people's bodies love yoga and walking. It's simply a matter of tuning into what nourishes your body.

    You can put together a group of different exercises that fit in with your daily moods or energy levels. If you feel unfocused, you could try vigorous activities like running or kickboxing. If you are feeling tight and tense, swimming or yoga is great. For some people, vigorous exercise might be a good idea when their energy levels are up and gentle exercise is more suitable when their body needs to do something relaxing.

3. **What suits your personality?** If you are an outgoing personality type and love to exercise in groups, you might enjoy team sports with a competitive side to them. Alternatively, you may find exercising with a buddy is inspiring and helps to keep you on track. If you are quiet and like to exercise alone, then walking and exercising near your home may suit you best.

4. **When do you feel most energetic?** Some people's bodies are ready to go at 6.00 am. Other people require food and gentle movement before exercising. However, I do recommend

incorporating a daily morning stretch routine into your exercise program. It can be just 10 minutes, yet it sets your spine and limbs up for a day spent sitting and doing mostly sedentary activities.

5.   **Think about the most convenient and easiest way to integrate exercise into your daily activity.** Convenience, ease and comfort are important. If I am busy and working hard, I swap my exercise regime to walking because I can do that anywhere and anytime from my home. Swimming takes about 1.5 hours out of my day, including travel to a pool. If a gym is your 'thing', look for one close to either your work or home. Gyms that are part of a franchise organisation may also have a branch in other locations you travel to.

It is important that you actually enjoy the type of exercise you do and not just do it because it is convenient. If convenience is the main driver for your exercise program, then you will probably tire of it and lose momentum. I don't go to gyms because I like to exercise outdoors. So make sure you are happy with where and what you are doing for exercise.

I see a lot of people walking and running with their dogs every day. This form of exercise may be convenient and enjoyable for you as well.

Experiment with different types of exercise and find what is best suited to your body, and what you enjoy doing. You will most likely find that you can then make it part of your daily nourishment.

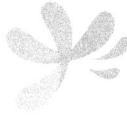

Chapter 11
Staying Motivated to Exercise

Motivation is the key to maintaining continuous movement and keeping yourself fit for a long, healthy life. Lack of motivation usually causes a slump in your exercise program so that you fall into an 'on/off' approach to exercise – rather like 'on/off' dieting patterns. In this chapter, I will discuss ways you can stay motivated to exercise and how to find your motivation again when you lose it.

Six Tips to Maintain your Motivation to Exercise

1. **Give yourself a head start on motivation:** I suggest you find some form of exercise that really suits your body, your lifestyle and your personality. Don't be swayed by advertising and other people's exercise programs that suggest that you have to go to the gym and throw a medicine ball around or run up 20 flights of stairs. If that isn't you, don't attempt to follow this advice. If it is you, then do the high-intensity cross training thing. You are unique and your body will thrive when you find the right type of movement for it.

2. **To stay motivated to exercise, keep it simple**: Do what you really enjoy; get instructions from your body as to what it needs in any given week or on the day. Tune into your moods and be prepared to 'fall off the wagon' on some occasions. Then, just get back on instead of beating yourself up.

3. **Strategise your exercise program**: Make the decision to do some kind of regular exercise that you actually like. Sit down and write out your exercise goal and post it in a prominent place, like your bathroom mirror or fridge. Set yourself up with a journal or exercise sheet (you can refer to the example exercise form that I've provided below) that outlines your exercise schedule for the week. If you like structure, create a campaign for up to three months in advance that is based on increasing your exercise levels in a way that fits in with your lifestyle.

A great way to stay motivated is to keep track of your exercise program. You can do this in any format that suits you, but here is a suggestion for an exercise form you might like to experiment with.

Example of an Exercise Form

Rule up a notebook or create a spreadsheet and set out the week days and types of exercise you are planning on doing. List the type of exercise along the vertical axis and the number of weeks along the horizontal axis. Record the type of exercise and the number of minutes you spend doing it.

Here is a simple example:

Type of exercise	Number of minutes Number of weeks				
	1	2	3	4	5

You can keep note of your weekly exercise schedule in whatever form you prefer. The trick is to do it regularly. It will definitely increase your motivation. Once you get into the groove with exercise and sort out a few other aspects of your health, everything will start to come together for you. You will feel so much better and your health and vitality will be on the rise.

1. **Inform friends and family of your commitment to your exercise regime:** Tell them in detail what you are going to do and write it down to keep yourself accountable. You could also find an exercise buddy who you can exercise with and/or get them to help you to keep on track, and vice versa.

2. **When you are not exercising, become a more active person:** It is a lot easier for you to achieve your exercise goals if you make the decision to become a physically active person – someone who sits less and moves more. There is growing amount of research which indicates that sitting too much is not good for us. We tend to sit at our jobs, to watch television, to eat, and so on. Some of the health issues related to sitting too much include increased blood pressure, elevated cholesterol, plus cardiovascular disease. It also places pressure on our internal organs.

3. **Develop your motivational muscle:** Whenever your motivation to exercise slips, don't get down on yourself – just start again.

Don't worry and think that you have gone backwards. You haven't. You are just building your motivation muscle and that takes persistence. If you stay with it, it is likely you will develop a level of motivation that will stay with you and increase. You will likely become self-motivated about your exercise as you grow into it. You will also become more protective of making sure other people, things, and events do not hijack your exercise on a regular basis.

There is so much you have to do to navigate your path to good health; it seems as though every day there is a new thing that either promises to make you incredibly healthy or is something that is going to ruin your health. I truly believe that the answer to improving your health and wellbeing is to simplify your life. Cut out those unnecessary things that seem to invade your 'time for you'. To make more time for you do things like batch cooking (get your family to help if possible), watch less television and refrain from checking social media all the time. Try to plan, sort, and chuck out what isn't working in your life and replace it with new and improved practices. If you do this, you will have so much more time to do all of the things you really want to do.

The Benefits of Exercise

If you are not exactly sure about the benefits of exercise, here is a list to remind you when you are feeling a bit wayward.

Exercise and movement:

- controls weight
- lowers blood pressure
- improves sleep
- aids digestion

- increases energy, and improves mood and quality of life
- reduces depression and anxiety
- improves balance, coordination and flexibility
- reduces risk of heart disease
- can prevent osteoporosis
- decreases inflammation
- improves immune system function.

PART THREE

Your Mindset

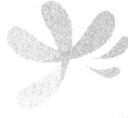

Chapter 12
A Great Mind

We are in the midst of a health revolution. Only fifteen years ago, the source of information about health would have been from your doctor, family and friends, and you would have been a passive recipient. Now, in a split second, we can research any type of health issue, diet, recipe, idea, application, or other advice via Google. More and more, we are learning ever-increasing amounts of information about all aspects of our health. We are gathering it, testing it, and going further with it in order to find the holy grail of health and wellbeing. At the same time, we are facing a huge global health crisis in terms of obesity and chronic illness.

The worldwide descent into obesity – first in the USA, then in Australia and many other countries in the West (and now also in Asia) – is one of the main motivators driving the upsurge of interest in health.

Mental health is a big part of this revolution. The concept and practice of mindfulness is now a major initiative in Australia and elsewhere. Ten years ago, when I attended a local yoga class, only those few people who were a bit 'alternative' were interested. Today, there is a yoga studio on every corner, and now meditation is catching on fast. We are rapidly embracing the notion of health as holistic, encompassing body, mind and spirit.

We have reached a tipping point where the combination of technology, motivation, and innovation are converging to create positive and profound influences for anyone who is looking to change their health and their life.

Underlying all of these recent changes is the principle that we are all unique and our individual health is dependent on us establishing a nutritional and lifestyle path that supports and relates to our uniqueness. And nothing is more unique than our own mind and emotions.

Some time ago, I had a boyfriend who astounded everyone because of his terrible diet and his subsequent enormous vitality. His daily intake of food and liquids included: 10–12 cans of Coca-Cola, half a bar of salami, a glass of chili juice, two 'normal' meals, one packet of cigarettes, and whatever else took his fancy. And yet he was the healthiest, most vibrant person I could have known. At the time, I always wondered how someone could eat and drink that stuff and still be so healthy. He was never sick – no colds, no anything – and he is still the same today.

The point of this story is not what he digested, but, rather, his attitude to what he digested.

He always enjoyed himself and never questioned anything he put in his mouth. He believed in himself more completely than anyone else I knew. He lived and digested all of the things about life that were in tune with his likes and general philosophy. He knew his own mind and acted in a way that completely supported his beliefs. You could say he was not in any conflict with himself and what he pursued in life.

In contrast, I have known many people who are so fixated on eating only the right food that this controls a large part of their daily lives. Not surprisingly, they often seem to be quite unhappy and not particularly well. People like this seem to spend all of their time thinking about, acting, planning and establishing ways to avoid eating things that contradict their philosophy of how they should eat. Clearly, if someone needs to eat a certain way or follow a specific diet for healing a disease or condition, then this is an exception. Sometimes we can go too far with fads; the supposed next new thing that will cure all of our woes. Do we become so appropriated by trends and mass marketing of food that we lose sight of what is really right for us?

During my studies to become a health coach, I learnt that Primary Health™ is more important than Secondary Health and these two scenarios highlight just what an important role our mind and emotions play in our health. Primary Health™, as defined by the Institute for Integrative Nutrition, refers to our lifestyle which includes our mental, emotional and spiritual health, as well as our relationships, engagement with exercise, and work. Secondary health is about what we digest and refers to the food and liquids we consume. When you put them all together – nutrition, exercise, body, mind, spirit, career and relationships – you get a fully-rounded picture of health and wellness. This is the revolution.

You may remember an action sequel in the film *The Matrix* that had a strong underlying message about the subliminal rules that dictate our lives. Joshua Rosenthal, Founder and Director of the Institute for Integrative Nutrition considers that we are completely surrounded and enveloped by a matrix that drains our life-force. According to Joshua 'it's a kind of mental, emotional, and spiritual programming'.[11]

Becoming truly healthy and happy requires you to follow a life journey that is defined by you for you. It is my experience that we have to rock our conditioning to avoid: staying in relationships that do us no good, working in a job that we don't love, and living our lives that do not honour our own uniqueness and force us to conform to social norms.

If we go against what is ultimately the right path for us, our health will suffer. Depression, anxiety, attention disorders, melancholy, and a form of 'zombiness' takes over and we become a desert within our own lives.

I challenge you to go gently towards the discomfort in your life. Try to examine your thoughts and look deeply into your life. Be honest with yourself and step-by-step move towards greater awareness. With increased awareness comes clarity, and clarity brings decisions, and decisions release the mud holding you down. And then, life supports your new decision.

The following suggestions will help you to get back in touch with your true self and look after your mind and emotions:

- Love and nurture yourself by doing things that nourish you.

- Pull your energy into yourself; hunker down inside yourself. Protect yourself from people, places, things, and events that don't nourish you.

- Be with people who nourish you – trusted friends, mentors, people who understand more about your life.

- Evaluate all of your commitments. Are they beneficial to your life? What don't you need anymore?

- Look at your relationship to stress and anxiety. Is this a common feature in your life?

- Adopt a slower pace in life. Walk slowly, eat slowly, and chew your food completely.

- Create realistic expectations of yourself and others.

- Have trust and faith that your life can and will change in accordance with your motivation and actions.

- Be vigilant with your time and who you spend it with.

- Take your attention away from your problems and get on with doing things in your life that move you forward.

- Take up meditation.

- Reach out to friends and loved ones. Connect with those people you love and care for.

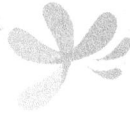

Chapter 13
Your Emotions and Attitude

What fires together, wires together.[12] This means that whatever we repeatedly think, do, experience, and feel will become a continual pattern in our life. It is only by consciously changing these patterns through a different mindset that we can be free of old habits and restrictions in our lives.

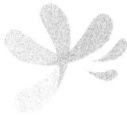

SHIFTING YOUR MINDSET – JANE'S STORY

Jane was a wonderfully accomplished person to the outside world. However, she was quite troubled on the inside. She was very skillful at disguising what was really going on in her life. In fact, to all outward appearances she seemed to be very much in control.

Jane suffered from lack of confidence when making decisions and being true to herself. She also didn't think that she deserved to have everything she wanted. She was quite anxious and insecure about her future, and she had a propensity to worry and to be fearful. Whenever challenges arose in her life she reverted to a negative way of thinking: this was the mindset or attitude that she adopted in all of her interactions with people, and was the filter through which she made decisions. It was no wonder that her life was not as she wanted when her mindset was preventing her from achieving the things she desired.

Her mother was like this as well and her behavior had a big influence on Jane being stuck in her life. She was intelligent enough to recognise the relationship of genetics to her own behavior, and she also knew that she was responsible for her life, and that her thoughts had a significant impact on her life. However, this was not a strong enough motivation for her to find a way to improve the situation. From a young age, her feelings of unworthiness had probably been hardwired into her brain. However, recent research into brain plasticity indicates that our brains can change over the course of our lifetime, growing new neural connections in remarkable ways.[13] As Jane got older, she started to see her life slipping away. Finally, as her life became 'a groundhog day' of unhappiness, it all became too much and she was forced to introspect to try to find an answer to her problems.

A voice inside her head said 'There must be more than this. How do I find it?' In that moment something clicked inside Jane and she changed her thinking. She earnestly questioned herself and the universe seeking an answer to her unhappiness. Jane's life began to change from that day forward. Help appeared in the form of an advertisement to sign up for a course in industrial design. She had always dreamed of doing further study but could never act on her dream because of her indecision.

Something had shifted in Jane. She was able to consider the opportunity from a different perspective – one of possibility rather than fear or self-doubt. Jane immediately enquired about a course of study and then applied to do something she had always wanted to do in her life. This one small act of courage started the ball rolling, and it was only the first step in transforming her life to be full of happiness and fulfillment.

Jane's story is familiar to us all in some way or another. Everyone has 'stuff' they are trying to deal with – that is what it is to be human. In our myopic way, we often tend to think we are worse off than others and that our lives have more challenges.

It is not what happens to you in life that defines you. It is how you deal with what happens to you that really matters.

The First Step to Inner Transformation

How do you develop a better understanding about the health of your mind and your emotions? It sounds like a complicated idea and a lot of hard work. My observations of people (and of myself) have highlighted to me that we spend a lot of time discussing and analysing everyone else's state of mind and emotional wellbeing, yet we rarely look at our own. We do this because we are able to see problems clearly in everyone else. It is much harder to recognise our own thoughts, feelings, and state of mind.

If you stop that process for a moment and concentrate on your thoughts and attitudes, you will be able to sort out a few things in your own 'internal cupboard'.

The first step is to understand what is 'firing together' and creating certain patterns in your life. Self-awareness is all-important because it brings clarity which, in turn, motivates you to try to change something in your life.

A few years ago, I spent a year learning how to use two fantastic tools for examining our thoughts and actions. They are contemplation and self-observation. These days, I use these two resources all the time in various ways; practicing and experimenting and making any changes I need to in my own life.

The Power of Contemplation

For good or for bad, all thought patterns become fixed or hardwired in our brains. Once these thought patterns are fixed, we form habits that keep them firmly in place. This is why changing our behavior to eat less junk food, stop smoking, remove ourselves from an abusive relationship, or an unhappy job can be so hard to do. Becoming more aware of our thinking and actions can be a very powerful tool to help us break the circuit of habitual thinking. This objective can be achieved by self-reflection or through contemplation which involves going within ourselves to reflect on our thoughts and actions in order to learn and grow from them.

No doubt you are familiar with the situation where you want to kick yourself for saying something that, on reflection, you are very sorry about. Yet, at the time, you just didn't seem to have control over your words. For example, you may be aware that you have a habit of finishing other people's sentences for them; it is something that you don't like doing but somehow you just keep doing it.

Activity

Take some time out from your usual routine and go into a quiet space away from people. Take a journal to jot down some thoughts as you start to practice a form of contemplation. Contemplation is a discipline that, like anything, the more it is practiced the more it benefits you, and the more you discover its value in your life.

Once you are in a quiet place, focus on quietening your mind and by turning your attention to your breathing, listening to your heartbeat, or to the sounds around you. If you are outside under a tree or in a garden, you can merely stare at a flower or an insect and let your mind focus on that for a while.

After a while as you notice that you have quietened your mind, you can turn your mind, you can turn your attention to thinking about what it is that you want to be, change or do differently in your life. This is not a thinking process; it is a focusing process whereby you simply allow thoughts to bubble up. It's a bit like identifying your intention to learn and grow from your reflection; just allow yourself to be and notice your thoughts. This is the act of going inwards, and it is a form of meditation.

As your mind starts to open up and you allow thoughts to freely come, you might like to jot them down. If you are used to journaling you might find that this practice leads to a flow of thoughts and reflections on yourself. Just go with it and let things come out and record them.

If you are new to this process, have patience and allow yourself to come back to it with a pure intent to learn the art of contemplation.

I follow this process when I mow the lawns, do the gardening or go for a walk. What fires together wires together: over the years I have created a nuronet for contemplation so it more or less comes naturally to me.

Contemplation will give you a different perspective on various aspects of your life. It can solve problems in your life by revealing a solution or a way to move on in some way. It is a beautiful process; it's sacred and often more valuable than paying someone to give you their perspective on your problems. This way you are able to tap into your own internal power to get your own solution. How good is that?

Let's look again at finishing other people's sentences. Let's say you have done some meaningful self-reflection and have some insight regarding how it feels to be with someone who isn't listening because they are too busy thinking about what they want to say. Let's say you have now realised that this is not how you want to be: instead you want to listen and talk from a new perspective. And to reinforce your decision, you post a note on your mirror or car dashboard so you can look at it often and start to form the new brain connections. You spend a few days further contemplating this, and then you let it go and see what happens.

Maybe this process works straight away for you. That's great. Or maybe you stumble and that's alright as well. As long as you keep going forward and stay with it, you will get results. And when you do get results, you will have an understanding that behavior change is possible and that you can do more of this by developing your 'muscle' of contemplation.

The Power of Self-Observation

In my understanding, the act of self-observation occurs when you become aware that you can hear your thoughts about yourself, hear yourself talking, or see yourself being – all from an observer's point of view. You are separated from the part of you that is caught up in the thinking or doing mode. This is different to self-reflection or contemplation. This is a powerful state of being in that you observe yourself in a moment saying or doing something you don't want to occur: you get an opportunity to turn off the drama in your mind as it happens because you are observing it rather than being it.

Hidden deep within us is the power to observe our own thoughts and actions. It is only hidden until we start to use this power and it is largely hidden because we almost always are 'being' our thoughts and emotions rather than observing them.

How can we 'be' and 'observe' ourselves at the same time?

This happens when you are doing or thinking something such as, 'I hate my body. It looks horrible' and you then are able to see or hear yourself saying or being this. In your mind you take a step back to observe this person who is yourself saying that they hate themselves. You literally separate from yourself and you watch yourself being so awful about you.

Another example is when you are having a fight with your partner or a friend and, in that moment, you step back and simply observe yourself speaking in a manner that later you would only regret.

The great potency of doing this in the moment is that you recognise that there is some other part of yourself that is able to separate out while you are doing something stupid, which we all do, and observe yourself in a detached manner. This is very powerful and, if you can do it a few times, it will help you to rewire what has been happening in your brain almost unconsciously. Then you can start to change what it is you want to think about your body, or indeed your life, or someone else.

Once you remove a pattern you don't want in your life, you are free to program whatever else you want in its place.

How to do an Audit on your Thoughts and Attitudes

Activity

Choose a day where you are able to focus and keep a journal in which you record your thoughts and attitudes from the moment that you wake in the morning to when you go to sleep at night.

Here are some suggestions you can follow to do a thought and attitude audit:

- Start the day with a quiet reflection or meditation about your intention for the day.

- From the moment you wake up, record your thoughts in your journal. A pocket–sized book is good so you can take it with you and have it at hand wherever you go throughout your day. For example, on the bus, at breaks, to the toilet, at lunch, going home, at home, and finally before bed. Regardless of whether you are working or not, whenever you get an insight into your thoughts, grab the journal and record it.

At the end of your day or on the following day, take a quiet half an hour to read through your journal. You could go into nature or somewhere else where you will not be disturbed. Read your written entries and reflect on what they mean to you.

Some questions you may want to ask yourself include:

- What keeps coming up for me?

- What am I thinking (that I may already know) but don't want to face?

- How do my thoughts and attitudes stack up against my values?

- What is positive about my thoughts?

- What would I like to do better or replace with something else?

If you do this with sincerity, it will be an act of self-love. We all have thoughts that are negative and positive. This exercise is about recognising where you are at in your life and deciding if there is anything you want to change about your attitudes and thoughts.

If you cannot see how you could change anything, that's ok too. This is a beginning of a process of clearing out what does not nourish you and substituting it with what does. It is a lifelong journey so it is best to take it at your own pace.

If and when you do the necessary work, the health and wellbeing of your mind and your body will be influenced positively. They are intimately connected and will respond favorably to your courage and action to nourish and love the greatness that dwells within you.

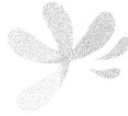

Chapter 14
How to do a Mind Cleanse

"A MIND THAT IS STRETCHED
BY NEW EXPERIENCES CAN NEVER
GO BACK TO ITS OLD DIMENSIONS."

– OLIVER WENDELL HOLMES, JR

In Chapter 13 we talked about identifying your dominant thoughts, and the emotional patterns and attitudes that are driving your decisions and experiences in life. In this chapter, I will discuss some additional activities that you can do in order to rid yourself of your mental and emotional baggage. These are not complicated practices and will make big inroads in helping you clear out the negativity in your life and replace it with the nourishing thoughts that will guide your life so it is inspired and purposeful.

The Early Morning Journal

This exercise was first devised by Julia Cameron who wrote *The Artist's Way*; a landmark book that has sold more than four million copies.[15] Her journaling program has been hugely successful and continues to help people find and develop their creativity in life.

Many of my clients use journaling to help them release negative 'baggage', old worn-out attitudes and beliefs that they don't need anymore. It works and is very effective for ridding your mind of destructive thought patterns.

Activity

Here is how this practice works. Buy or use a journal that you will use for this purpose alone. This is your private daily practice that will guide and nourish you as you chart your way through the challenging aspects of your current life. If that statement doesn't make sense now, it will once you have begun to empty your mind onto the page every day.

The key to morning journaling is to get up early so that you have sufficient time to write before the day gets underway.

Before you start your day, either sit up in bed or go to your writing space, open the page of your journal and immediately write the first thing that comes to mind. Just keep going with this, allowing your thoughts to empty out on the page. Fill up two A4 pages or three or four A5 pages. You will know when to stop. Just flow with it until it seems finished. All up, you should spend no longer than 20–30 minutes writing.

The trick is to not stop; just keep the flow coming onto the page and don't worry about what is coming out. If you feel blocked, just write anything – even a Dr Seuss rhyme will do. Just keep the momentum going and do what you intend to do. Don't analyse or have any expectations. JUST DO IT.

Commit to this exercise for at least two weeks. When you are no longer recording all of your woes, all of your problems and all of the other 'stuff', you have reached the end of the process. Another indication that you have managed to empty out all of your problems is that your writing changes to more positive thoughts.

Of course, you can continue writing whatever you like. When I first wrote my pages there was stuff that came out that shocked me, but I didn't judge it or try to stop it flowing – I just let it come. To this day, I have never gone back and reread what I wrote during that time. My journal is hidden among my other belongings and I really don't have any interest in reading about things that are no longer part of my life. Try this for yourself – I can guarantee that it works.

Gratitude

This is wonderful exercise that will help you to dissociate from living your life as a daily chore. Every evening before you go to sleep, write down three things you are grateful for during that day. No matter how small or large they may be, commit yourself to writing down three things. You might also like to write some details about each of them – not just simply: 'felt grateful for the apple my colleague gave me'. Add some more information such as: 'I was surprised and delighted by the apple that Sandra gave to me today. I had no morning tea and the act of giving me the apple prompted me to bring some in and keep them on my desk for others. I was so grateful for Sandra's thoughtfulness today'.

The act of doing this transforms your attitude towards everything in your life. Having an embedded attitude of gratitude for the things that happen to you on a daily basis will lift your spirits and put a spring in your step. All of us fall into patterns of drudgery and negativity, so you can be confident that other people will benefit if you adopt a daily gratitude practice. This, in turn, will transform the flow of energy between you and others in many surprising ways. Just think about how you feel when you meet someone who has a beautiful mind. It rubs off on you, doesn't it? If you follow this process regularly, your life will become graceful so that you become happier and shine.

Do this for one week and see what happens. If you discover that you love doing it and that it makes a difference in your life, then continue on with it.

There are many things you can do to uplift your life and create a great and beautiful mind.

Meditate

Meditation is becoming increasingly popular and many people are finding it very beneficial in their lives. There are many ways to meditate: if you have time you might like to do a course, or you may prefer to simply experiment with different ways of meditating yourself.

- Walking can be very meditative if you are able to bring your mind into the present moment and be centred in the environment around you.

- A guided meditation is a great way to start, either with someone who takes you through the process or via online or recording. You just have to watch out that you don't fall asleep too quickly. Don't worry if you do the first couple of times you meditate. As you continue this practice, you will find that your need for sleep diminishes and you shift to a profound sense of connection to the words as you follow them.

- If you are busy and are able to switch off relatively easily, you can do a quick five-minute meditation during lunch time. With meditation, it is not how long you sit there for; it is all about the quality of your focus when you do it. Five minutes of meditation can take away a problem at work, a tension, tiredness, or sadness. With experience, these quick meditations become more beneficial. Try it yourself and see what happens.

A good way to start your meditation is to sit up straight, cross-legged on a cushion or on a hard-backed chair with your feet on the floor. Close your eyes and take three to six deep diaphragm breaths and fill your body and head with oxygen. From here, you can mediate on something specific or on just being present in that space.

I recommend that you read and investigate meditation further and find out what suits you. You can experiment with different types and even make up your own version of meditation.

PART FOUR

Your Spiritual Wellbeing

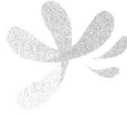

Chapter 15
Enlightened Spirit

"I CONSIDER MYSELF A STAINED-GLASS WINDOW. AND THIS IS HOW
I LIVE MY LIFE. CLOSING NO DOORS AND COVERING NO WINDOWS;
I AM THE MULTI-COLORED GLASS WITH LIGHT FILTERING THROUGH
ME, IN MANY DIFFERENT SHADES. ALLOWING LIGHT TO SHED AND
FALL INTO MANY HUES. MY JOB IS NOT TO DIRECT ANYTHING,
BUT ONLY TO FILTER INTO MANY COLORS. MY ANSWER IS
DESTINY AND MY GUIDE IS JOY. AND THERE YOU HAVE ME."

- C. JOYBELL C.

In this chapter, I offer a way to deepen your connection with yourself, and to expand your knowledge so you can be your own resource for a healthy body and life. It all matters: every part of your life plays a role in your overall health.

As part of our busy lives, we are continually immersed in an environment of hyper-connectivity via a range of different digital technologies which have many advantages; however, we are rapidly finding it difficult to contain its role in our lives.

Unlike previous generations who had close ties to the natural world, the rapid growth of digital technology has meant that we have become much less connected to nature.

Spirit and spirituality are different concepts for each of us. You may have a faith-based spirituality, or some other form. Your spirituality may be simply an appreciation of being alive, or it may be that you combine your chosen religion with your own form of spirituality. Maybe your connection with Spirit comes from being in nature, or through meditation. Maybe you don't really know what your vision of spirituality involves, but what you do know is that some things in life move you to tears of joy, or that you feel a shiver up your spine when someone tells you a remarkable story where someone has triumphed over incredible adversity.

I don't think anyone can absolutely define 'spirit' because it is a very personal thing, and is different for all of us.

The important thing is that your relationship with spirituality is yours alone to develop in whatever way brings meaning, understanding and peace to your life.

My personal belief is that I am part spirit, part matter, and part soul. For the majority of my life, I have sought to feel my Spirit more and make a connection with it in order to know it better. For many years, I have searched for answers to all the big questions about life. I have incorporated meditation as a daily practice in my life. I view all of my life as spiritual – not just the so-called spiritual activities but every aspect of life. And my greatest teacher has always been nature. I have been extraordinarily fortunate to be able to spend long periods of time in nature to observe, reflect and learn.

Spirituality can be practical and visceral in the way we act and relate to all living things. It's not' 'woo woo'. Instead, it's a grounded and practical vital force; a way of finding your own personal truth about life.

There have been times in my life when I've felt completely lost, and it is during these periods that I would escape to be within nature. Sometimes this would simply consist of a walk or retreat for a few days; other times it was a pilgrimage into the wilderness. My biggest trip involved a mostly solo journey into the Canadian Arctic to trek and immerse myself in the experience of nature. As I travelled through Arctic tundra and treeless mountain landscape, I found that my fear fell away and I became more in tune with everything around me. It was as though nature was cleansing my mind and my body so that I was able to think much more clearly about what was really important about life – and about my life in particular.

During my Canadian expedition, I drove along the Dempster Highway, which was mostly graded dirt, and passed through large areas of the Arctic wilderness. One day I came across a mountain and was drawn to climb it. As I set out, I had one question in my mind – to gain a clear understanding about which path to take in my life at a time when I was unclear. Without knowing anything about the view at the top, I headed upward and when I reached the peak of this mountain I found myself looking to the right at a massive range of jagged mountains called the Northern Cordilleran Volcanic Province and to the left an older, rounded basin. I was looking directly at two distinct geological epochs – the Miocene and the Holocene. Yet, the geology is not what was significant to me in that moment.

What I observed was Nature reflecting my two paths. A flatter, rounded basin blended into a dynamic stretch of jagged mountains as far as I could see. This was a direct visual representation to me of the paths of nature on a huge scale, corresponding to my current choices in life. I sat and reflected on what it all meant. I left that mountain with clear knowledge of my path.

What caused those two different geological formations to have what I call a 'connection impact' on me?

I had climbed this mountain with an intention to resolve the dilemma in my mind about alternate pathways in my life, and when I reached the top it was as though the natural world was mirroring my thoughts and allowing me to find clarity. Was nature doing this in reality? At this point it really doesn't matter. The important thing is that what occurred during that mountain climb made the experience unforgettable for me and as a result the decision I made was extremely powerful.

Nature can have a magical quality that you can tap into. It can provide you with clarity of mind when you go deeply into its fold. Sometimes nature mirrors you so you get to experience a remarkable unspoken connection. You will always discover something about yourself when you immerse yourself in nature with the intention to grow and learn.

Connecting with your Spirit or Source to Guide You

You can actively tap into and allow your spirit to help guide you through life. It can be like your internal best friend. I achieve this through contemplation and self-observation as I explained in Chapter 13. I often choose to contemplate important things when I am walking, gardening, or just sitting in the sun in the backyard. I go deep into nature when I want to renew my spirit and attitude to life. I have found this approach to have a profoundly powerful impact on my life.

Sometimes you can do this especially if you are bluntly reminded that I need to slow down and become present again, especially if I am under pressure and busy. Learning to be present in the moment is important and it is a work-in-progress for those of us who desire the benefits of this experience. I am pleased that meditation and mindfulness are reaching more lives today. It is a sign that we have a deep need for these spiritual techniques in our lives.

You may have a connection with your Spirit while listening to uplifting music, or when something extraordinary happens in life in which the expression of love triumphs over fear or adversity. We often get a shiver up our spine, or the hairs stand up on our arms. In my opinion, this is an indication of a connection with our source or our Spirit.

Perhaps Spirit is the opposite to ego, which is concerned more about survival: we need both to guide us. I have noticed that the Spirit is quieter than the ego, and we have to make a concerted effort to allow it into our life when the ego and personality get a bit out of control.

Activity to Reflect on

What does the term 'spirit' mean to you?

This is very personal question so I suggest that you devote some time thinking about your relationship with that side of yourself. Meditation is a definite technique to be able to tune into that side, and be at one with it.

Another activity is to write some words to describe what the term spirit means to you. Before doing so, close your eyes and breathe deeply to feel your mind and body become aligned; empty your mind from all thoughts about doing this or that. Just breathe and be in the present moment. When you feel calm and relaxed, write your thoughts about Spirit and what it means to you.

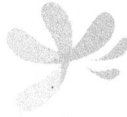

Chapter 16
The Link Between People and Nature

I find truth in Einstein's quote. But it also brings up the question of what will happen when there is no healthy nature to look deep into?

This chapter is a slight departure from discussing high-achieving women's health. Instead, I have explored how our physical, mental and emotional health is dependent upon nature. I would love this chapter to prompt you to question how your interest in health could be a key to valuing nature more.

For more than 25 years, I worked in the area of environmental sustainability. My role spanned Australia and overseas, advising governments and communities on how to repair degraded rivers and soils, and plant more trees. I transitioned my career to human health because I had become disheartened witnessing too many cuts to the health of the environment and not enough improvements.

Just before my career change, I was responsible for the development of a ten-year sustainability strategy for a rural region in Australia. Through talking to communities at all levels, my team learned of the link between the health of the environment and human health. For the first time in the field of environmental planning we forged a concrete link between the creation of resilient agricultural landscapes and resilient communities; the common denominator being that healthy and resilient environments equate to healthy and resilient people. This work also extends to socio-economic health.

One example of these links is the effect of environmental pollutants such as heavy metals, pesticides, herbicides and chemicals in and on our foods. The increased toxicity levels in our foods, such as mercury in fish, and large industrialised farming methods are likely contributors to the growing problem of poor health. The jury is still out on the impact of toxic chemicals in our food systems; however, eating organic or spray-free food is a choice more and more people are making everyday because they consider it is better for their health.

The leading cause of illness and death in Australia is chronic health conditions. Although we are living longer, we are increasingly living with debilitating lifestyle diseases such as diabetes, autoimmune disease, and serious digestive conditions.[16] Many chronic health conditions can be prevented or reversed with restorative health measures that help the body to heal itself. Functional nutrition, or specific types of food, can play a critical role in the repair and the proper functioning of our bodies.

Why are lifestyle diseases the leading cause of death and illness in Australia? We all know that poor diet and stress play a significant role. For example, the clients I see in my practice all suffer from symptoms caused by ingesting gluten from wheat. Some are serious and others less serious. I don't let the divided research on this subject determine whether they would fare better with or without gluten – I let their bodies be the judge. After eliminating gluten from their diets, 100 per cent of my clients report an improvement in their wellbeing and energy levels.

Why are so many of us becoming sensitive to eating gluten? One possible reason is that, as a result of technological advances in agriculture, we have modified the wheat plant to such an extent that our bodies have decreased ability to digest wheat. For some of you, removing gluten for a time will give your body a chance to recover so that you may be able to tolerate it later in much smaller quantities. For others more sensitive, it will be best to leave gluten out all together. Again, because we are all unique, each of our situations will vary.

What about our soil? If the soil we grow food in declines in quality, the nutrient content and value of the food we eat also declines and has an impact on our health in some way. Much of Australia's broadacre farming has soil which is depleted and contains too little organic matter to be able to provide the essential nutrients and minerals for producing healthy plants. The farmer adds those minerals using chemical fertilisers rather than through building healthy soil. This situation is slowly changing because of our greater knowledge and understanding about soil health, but it will take a long time to rebuild Australia's depleted soils that were not very robust from the start.

According to the Australian Institute of Health and Welfare, our busy 21st century lives are largely the cause of the decline of our general health. Even though we don't yet know all the answers, we need to pay heed to the precautionary principle where we take action when we see the signs, rather than waiting for the conclusive scientific evidence when it is often too late.

I wonder: could our actions to heal ourselves facilitate a role for us in healing the Earth? I believe that as we strive to heal our bodies we become more aware of how polluted food, toxic cleaning substances and cosmetics, and poor lifestyle choices are all contributing to our poor health. We will begin to feel the impact of these factors more personally as we make healthier choices to crowd out the toxic choices. We've all seen people who have the realisation of the connections between their health and the source of their foods; over time they become advocates for a healthier environment for themselves and their families, and even their communities.

So what can we do to act on our understanding of the link between the environment's health and our own health? To help nature and ourselves, we can grow our own food. Consuming food that other people have grown thousands of miles away is far less physically and mentally healthy than growing our own. We can also stop using harmful cleaning solutions in our homes. Using vinegar and bicarbonate soda to clean our homes does the same job without harming the earth's waterways.

Small actions for our health and our environment can turn into significant changes in our lives. A greater connection to nature is good for our health – mentally, spiritually, and physically.

We need to 'develop an interest in what influences' our body's health, our organs, and the way our physiological systems work as a whole so we can make informed choices and see the links between our overall health and the health of the environment.

For example, our contemporary lifestyles mean that our livers are under far more pressure and can only cope with processing and eliminating a certain amount of toxins before the increased levels start to build up and become absorbed back into our body. This is when illness can occur. It is likely that the health of our planet is somewhat similar in that the more we keep damaging the planet, the more the problems back up and natural systems begin to weaken.

As we continue to experience toxic physical and mental conditions in our daily lives, we are forced to take stock. This situation has arisen quite suddenly in our evolution. For thousands of years we lived in connection with nature and conducted our farming practices in a natural way. Then, in less than 100 years, we have dramatically changed everything. We have traded the perceived freedom of readily available produce in any season for a toxic industrialised farming system. We need to remember that we are intelligent beings who always have choices in the steps we take, including the way we farm on a large scale.

At this point, our collective health and the health of the planet are both going backwards in a serious way. Perhaps this outlook can only be explained by what a good friend of mine once said: 'Humans are great at fixing problems but terrible at preventing them.'

Reconnecting with nature

Thinking about Einstein's quote, one of the best things you can do for your own health is to go into a natural environment to experience and develop an understanding that is deeply personal to you.

Next time you find yourself in nature:

- Spend some time just observing what links you to the natural world around you.

- Think about your body and life as a natural landscape or system that all works harmoniously when it is properly cared for, and can turn to chaos when a few things start to go wrong. How do you view this in light of my discussion about nature? Do you consider that some parts of your life are thriving whereas other parts are wilting? Are those parts that are suffering due to the fact that you have not properly cared for them? And what possible role do toxins in your environment play in the health of your body, both from a mental and physical health standpoint?

- To lighten things up, you could take your journal into nature and write your musings or a poem that reflects your thoughts.

Focus on the wonderful things about your life that you may have forgotten about.

You might want to also think about the health of your family and ways you can influence them to make small changes in the same way that you are doing. We can all be educators when we have knowledge.

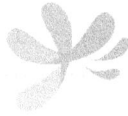

Chapter 17
Self-Discovery through Nature

Nature is with you everywhere: the trees and grass in your backyard; your veggie patch; the park just down the road; the night sky with the moon and stars; and the mountain walk that is a short drive away. It's present in many forms, there for you to make a connection.

Human interaction with the natural world has been a major part of our lives and our development for thousands of years. Only in very recent times – since the Industrial Revolution – have we started to drift away. During the past 100 years, our cities and towns have become increasingly electrified, and in the last 20 years mobile phones and wireless devices have almost become a symbiotic part of us.

When we are connected to the earth and nature, we experience a feeling of being centered, balanced and anchored in the flow of this energy. And it is becoming increasingly obvious that, with the fast pace of our digital, electrified world, we need to be able to tap into this healing, life-affirming energy in our lives.

Why is Nature Beneficial?

Nature is grounding, non-judgmental, uplifting, and calming. It is also violent, destructive and powerful. Nature can reflect wisdom and knowledge back to us, and allow us to learn from it. To enjoy the benefits, you can choose to go into nature in a small way – or in a big way. If you go there with the intention of discovering and learning about yourself, much will be revealed to you.

Recently, I have been visiting my local park which has a beautiful natural watercourse running along its border. I walk along the path, peer into the tree-lined riverbed with its large rocks, and watch as the water tumbles across the rocks and then continues on its way. The steep banks are lined with exotic weeds, but even those are doing their job by holding the surrounding soil in place.

This park is home to many birds and butterflies, and it creates a wonderfully cooling atmosphere for the joggers who use the path in the mornings and afternoons. I love to just be there and absorb into my being the journey of the river when it waits silently for rain and when it rushes by after a rainfall. I observe a feeling of peacefulness about this area. People are exercising, walking or just sitting on the field nearby. It is like we are all grounded; made 'real' again by this environment without knowing why or how.

Does this experience of being in nature and absorbing its beauty and peace resonate with you?

Simple Ways to Connect with Nature at Home

To become grounded with the earth you can go outside and walk on the grass with bare feet. Doing this regularly will bring you a sense of peace and help you to feel balanced and centered.

You can also go outside just before bed and look up at the night sky; it will bring you back to a feeling of connectedness with nature. You might feel awe at the size of the moon or at the brightness of the stars. The act of simply spending five minutes to look up at our universe and check how immeasurable it is, reminds us that there is more to our lives than petty things – there is vast opportunity for all of us right here and now.

Walking for Pleasure

I have always enjoyed walking. I have bushwalked in Australia, Canada, New Zealand, and other places. I have sometimes felt extremely challenged by nature and pushed to overcome misery, fatigue, pain and danger.

This is not necessarily an activity that everyone wants to be involved in, but I often sought out adventure and challenges with its corresponding feelings of danger and risk. In all of those experiences, I grew as a person and developed a deeper understanding of life and nature.

A study conducted by researchers at the University of Michigan found that walking in a group within nature has multiple health benefits, including an improvement in mood, decreased depression, enhanced wellbeing and mental health, and lower levels of stress. The effects on mood seem to be particularly beneficial to people who have experienced a traumatic life event, such as the loss of a loved one or a divorce.

According to Sara Warber, Associate Professor of Family Medicine at the University of Michigan Medical School: 'Walking is an inexpensive, low risk and accessible form of exercise and it turns out that combined with nature and group settings, it may be a very powerful, under-utilised stress buster. Our findings suggest that something as simple as joining an outdoor walking group may not only improve someone's daily positive emotions but may also contribute a non-pharmacological approach to serious conditions like depression'.[17]

Likewise, an article in *The Huffington Post* about the health benefits of walking reveals that it can lead to better cardiovascular health, reduced stress, improved mood and self-esteem, healthy weight, strengthened bones, and a boost in creative thinking.[18]

Rediscovering Wild Nature

Beyond our backyards, local city parks and recreation areas is wild nature which offers something quite different to a cultivated parkland experience. In their book *The Rediscovery of the Wild*, Peter H. Khan Jnr. and Patricia H. Hasbach suggest that 'Wildness often involves that which is big, untamed, unmanaged, not encompassed, and self organising, and unencumbered and unmediated by technical artifice. We can love the wild, we can fear it. We are strengthened and nurtured by it.'[19]

As a child, I grew up wild in fringes of the country town of Castlemaine in Victoria. My brother was ten years older than me and I looked up to him. He would heave me over the back fence and we would take off through the local foundry to seek out our next discovery in nature. This sometimes involved digging underground tunnels and sometimes exploring disused gold mines, but it was always an adventure. I remember one time crawling like rabbits through a tunnel that was under the railway line. From these days I developed my yearning for adventure and freedom, and I developed a level of respect and connection with nature which would continue to have a grounding and powerful influence in my life.

Later, these childhood experiences led me to live in one of Australia's great wild places in the Northern Territory of Australia, Cobourg Peninsula, which is also named Garig Gunak Barlu National Park, and is home to several groups of Aboriginal traditional owners. We hunted in bare feet, ate what we caught, and lived in a tiny community that consisted of a couple of families. It was a life connected with nature on all levels. There was wildlife galore all around us – crocodiles, buffalo, wild banteng, oceans, rainforests, coral reefs, and plenty of things to do in nature.

These days within my health practice, I help women to reconnect with nature – both tame and wild. I consider it to be an experience we are all yearning for, but are unaware we are missing. It offers the freedom to be wild and unfettered by our contemporary urban lifestyle; the freedom to experience what we have lost with the advent of technological progress and industrialisation. For the most part, wild places have become a rarity on this planet.

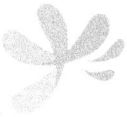

APPRECIATING WILDERNESS AREAS – GILL'S STORY

A good friend of mine recently shared her story of her love of wild and remote places with me. Gill has spent much of her working life looking after wilderness and natural places in Australia. She and her husband, Peter have undertaken walks in almost every corner of the world, in some of the most beautiful, untouched and challenging places imaginable.

Most of Gill's walks have been in mountainous regions and often for up to 15 days at any one time.

For Gill and Peter, walking was initially about experiencing and understanding the natural environment, particularly in Australia and New Zealand. Later, they ventured to great wilderness regions such as Patagonia, Alaska, the Himalayas and the John Muir trail in California. Over the years, their walking passion grew to include walking to combine nature and culture in such places as Bhutan, Nepal and many parts of Europe. According to Gill, 'There is nothing better than walking into a remote village and experiencing the people and their daily lives as you find them'.

I really wanted to understand what a lifetime of walking meant for Gill, so I called her and had a lively conversation that made me want to grab my boots and pack my bag. She described it as being able to get away from the demands of life such as other people, work, maintaining a house and garden, cars, and the digital world.

In Gill's words: *'Our lives are the complete opposite of nature; they are stressful and demanding all the time. I love walking in the wildness without any of the usual daily judgments, complexity, anxiety, and stress. The incredible beauty and variety of the landscape is both a spiritual and rejuvenating experience that is hard to describe.*

I love the solitude and meditative experience of walking. You seem to develop a rhythm and all the noise in your head gets turned off. I feel safe knowing that Peter is up ahead and that I am alone but not really alone. I always come away feeling a strong sense of peace. I also love not having to put on appearances. I can walk in my shorts, T shirt – unshowered and dishevelled, never feeling judged by nature. I feel incredibly self-sufficient when I am walking. Knowing that life is simple and that every base is covered enables me to feel very much at home in nature.

I also love the challenges that wild places offer. I find them rejuvenating – both mentally and physically – and I love feeling tired at the end of a full day of walking. It's such a healthy kind of tiredness. I get a growing sense of freedom every time I do a walk.

One of the most important things I have learnt over the years is to never underestimate the importance of fresh unpolluted water and clean mountain air.

Walking in the wilderness isn't always fun. I have experienced debilitating fear, especially when getting caught in dangerous thunderstorms and having to traverse rocky slopes. Although really frightening, it has taught me what triggers fear in me and how to deal with it. I understand anxiety and how to watch it, and to think rationally about it.'

I guess we cannot spend all of our lives travelling the world to walk in the great wilderness, and other natural and cultural areas, but we can certainly experience it in a way that is right for us. And, at the same time, we can witness life from a new perspective and feel rejuvenated without paying exorbitant prices for a retreat.

We can rediscover the wildness that lives within ourselves – scary as it might seem to do that. The rewards will always stay with us and help us to improve our lives by connecting with the supportive and nurturing force of nature.

Contemplating in Nature

As I mentioned previously in Chapter 13, contemplation is the act of going within yourself to consider an idea, concept, decision or way of understanding something. Contemplating in nature is very powerful. Simply finding a comfortable rock to sit on, or a tree to lean against, or just getting into the rhythm of a walk can be beneficial. It is best to go into nature with no forms of distraction on you, such as mobile phones.

As a general guide, you can practise the act of contemplation in the following way:

Ask yourself a question. That question can be anything you want to clarify, understand or receive an answer for. The strength of your intent will determine how much value you get from your contemplation. If you really desire something to be revealed to you, then you will get the answer.

The act of asking a question and contemplation are two quite different things. You can ask the question by saying it out aloud to yourself, or writing it down, or even by just asking it in your head. In contrast, contemplation involves becoming quiet within, stopping your thinking process and simply focusing on something in nature; a flower, a tree and blade of grass will do. You can also just focus on listening to the birds. The idea is to go into a light trance. Don't worry about snakes or any wildlife affecting you; they won't bother you if you are not tromping around threatening their world.

If you look at something in nature with an empty mind you will find that contemplation will come readily to you. It is like a muscle; the more you use it, the easier it becomes to do.

Exploring within Nature

Exploring within nature is intriguing. Sometimes it's good to go micro and look at insects, patterns on trees, fungi or whatever. Other times it is great to find a high point with a vista looking out over the horizon to watch birds and just immerse yourself in the view. I find if you go with someone else, it becomes a talk-walk fest and you miss out on experiencing everything around you. It can be good to do a hike with someone where you put a bit of distance between yourselves and then catch up again throughout the day.

Other Ideas that Connect You with Nature

You might like to take up nature photography, drawing, writing prose or poetry. Capture your experiences and then write about them when you are back at home. Find a project in nature. It could be to document all of the birds you see or listen to bird calls and identify what birds they are by their calls. Building a herb or veggie garden is also a good way to connect with the soil and the growth of plants. Growing food is marvellous because it provides the best form of nutrition when you pick the produce just before using it. The act of growing food is also about creating something that nourishes you.

Nature is an abundant source of life and it is a great place to exercise your brain. Get into it!

PART FIVE

Your Work and Career

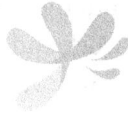

Chapter 18
Are You Happy in Your Work?

"WHEN YOU ARE INSPIRED BY SOME GREAT PURPOSE, SOME
EXTRAORDINARY PROJECT, ALL YOUR THOUGHTS BREAK
THEIR BOUNDS. YOUR MIND TRANSCENDS LIMITATIONS,
YOUR CONSCIOUSNESS EXPANDS IN EVERY DIRECTION AND
YOU FIND YOURSELF IN A NEW, GREAT AND WONDERFUL
WORLD. DORMANT FORCES, FACULTIES AND TALENTS BECOME
ALIVE, AND YOU DISCOVER YOURSELF TO BE A GREATER
PERSON BY FAR THAN YOU EVER DREAMED YOURSELF TO BE."

– PATANJALI

Most of us spend a great deal of our precious time at work – much
more than we spend sleeping or doing anything else. So what a waste
of time it is if we are not happy there. Do you work just because that's
your sustenance, or do you work for something you believe in and

genuinely love? I meet a lot of people from all walks of life who are not glowing with happiness about their work. In fact, they are often so consumed by the demands of work and of their lives that it is hard for them to be glowing about anything. When did we get confused about what work is? And when did we agree to settle for a job that really doesn't suit us?

It's very difficult to get off the 'hamster wheel' of unsatisfactory work. Many people feel trapped working in jobs that do not really fit with who they are, or in positions where their valuable skills are not contributing to the world. Their tolerance for the discomfort zone and their attitude to change will determine whether they will face the tough choice to either leave a job they don't love, or try to change it from within their organisation. Sometimes they are just too scared to follow a passion, so they convince themselves that it couldn't possibly work out if they tried.

I love helping women to build a healthy and productive life that is sustainable, rather than a productive life that causes them to feel burnt out and stressed. Being unsatisfied in your work can definitely lead to a range of health problems including stress; depression; anxiety; mood disorders such as irritability, negativity and sadness; and bad eating habits such as snacking on sugary foods or drinking too much alcohol. You can also get into conflict more easily with co-workers and with family members and friends when you are not happy at work. And you can ultimately become a dull dissatisfied person who is just going through the motions of life.

You also need to look at your level of satisfaction with your work and recognise that if you are not happy with this aspect of your life your health will suffer. This is because your mental and emotional state has a significant impact on your physical health.

You may not be aware of what your life passion is and where your strengths lie. Maybe you are a generalist and are highly capable at anything. This can make it even more challenging to find a particular focus given that you might enjoy doing many different things.

Maybe you don't have the courage to pursue the things you really want to do in your life. Or are they buried too deep for you to clearly see what they are? You may be in a bit of a fog and low in energy, so passion and purpose feel unattainable. Often, if you address the problem of low energy, you can think more clearly about finding happiness through your work.

Recently, one of my clients was feeling very low in energy and was experiencing a number of other debilitating physical health conditions. Once I had helped her to build up her energy levels and worked on her other health issues, she had sufficient mental energy and interest to start planning out her work and the rest of her life. She was also able to take logical steps towards moving out of her current job into a field that she loved, and that inspired her. She saw new possibilities and ways in which she could reach her goals. This was not available to her before she'd addressed her physical health issues.

Of course, there are those other lucky people who seem to hit the ground running, fully aligned with their purpose and desires. They see what they want to do and how they can contribute with a great deal of clarity. It's easy to envy those people. However, everyone's journey is unique to them and we each are here in the world to do things our way and to make our own valuable contribution.

Some of us are keen to experience a number of careers, work options, and loves. We have to be courageous to follow this path as it usually means a lot of change in our lives.

I have learnt over the years that it helps to have a clear idea of your values and what feels right for you. It is important not to simply do what seems right for others, especially due to perceived (or otherwise) pressure from friends and family.

Reflecting on Career Choices

Are you at a stage where a large part of your life is already behind you? Has it just dawned on you that there is something else in life in store for you? You might find yourself at a crossroad in your career – an uncomfortable time when you need to work out what you actually want to do. You may be wondering and waiting for something to happen. But nothing will without your input; you have to do something. You will be searching for answers and questioning yourself: Could I? What if? Am I good enough? What about the money?

There are no right or wrong answers. I believe that the best approach is to take the necessary time to reflect and ask yourself what really matters to you. Sometimes you just have to have the courage to start the conversation with yourself. Will you be happier and healthier if you move away from your past 10–15 years of work? You can also ask a trusted friend to help you to talk through your thoughts about your work or find a career coach who can advise you.

So if you find yourself wondering about that 'one other thing', that 'sliding door' that you could have walked through, it's time to give it some credence. Allow yourself to at least think about it with an open mind in order to consider the possibilities for change. How do you feel when you think about it? How long have you been thinking about it? What would happen if you were to change direction in your work life?

Ideas for Transition in your Life

There's always a bridge of transition between where you are and where you want to be in life. You may simply need to brush up on your resume and apply for other jobs. You may need to invest in another qualification that will lead you to a new career or promotion.

One of the best things you can do is to invest in yourself. You are an asset for your future, so if you don't invest in yourself you narrow your opportunities and there are fewer choices open for you in the world.

Don't worry about what stage of life you are in or what your circumstances are. Simply try to become clear about what you want in your career and your life. Question what being alive means to you and then make a plan for how you might be able to do the work you really love. Step-by-step, you can develop a way to be happier and more inspired about the work you do. You just have to make a start and develop a strategy to go forward with.

We live in exciting times. It's a golden era for women to be able to step up to their purpose on this planet – boldly, courageously, and with a wild heart. You can feel like you did when you were younger, but with the benefit of wisdom that comes with age and experience.

If you feel as though you have something more to do in your life, no matter what your current age is, aim to do it if you can. Find a way that works for you. If you are unhappy in your work, it will have a negative impact on your health. Only you can decide what is your real priority – good health or unsatisfactory work.

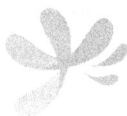

Chapter 19
The Demons of Fear

There is a well-known book by Susan Jeffers, PhD called *Feel the Fear and Do it Anyway*. This is an excellent book if you want to find out how to deal with the things you most fear, or how to learn how to be more comfortable with fear.

I love the Lord of the Rings books and films for many reasons; a primary one being the various ways that the characters overcome fear. There is a great scene in the first Lord of the Rings film *The Fellowship of the Ring* when the wizard, Gandalf the Grey is stranded on one side of a bridge facing the huge fiery monster Balrog, while his friends have made it to the other side. Gandalf stands on the bridge – a tiny figure in comparison to the monster. He summons up all his authentic power to fiercely say to the Balrog, 'You shall not pass'. With all his might, he strikes the bridge with his sword and the bridge crumbles in front of him. The Balrog falls and tumbles to his death. For a moment, everything seems to be over, until the Balrog sends a whip of fire up to hook Gandalf and drag him down as well. Gandalf descends into the abyss while fighting this fiery creature all the way down; never giving up the fight until he finally conquers it. In the end, he does manage to conquer the Balrog and then he transforms into Gandalf the White – a more powerful wizard than he was previously.

Gandolf didn't stop to wonder or work out if he could achieve this brave feat. In his heart, he knew that this was what he had to do.

This scene in the *The Fellowship of the Ring* film is a metaphor for all the demons of fear that stop us all from pursuing our dreams. Obviously, it is magnified for dramatic effect in this story; however, it does send a strong message to us about overcoming our demons of fear in order to emerge triumphant and more powerful than before.

You can use this metaphor and story to remind you about what you do not want to occur in your life. If you want to change your life in some way, you may need to summon all of your power to cross that bridge and meet the challenge. You have to believe in something that you cannot yet see or touch. You have to believe in yourself and your ability to reach your goals.

Fear comes in all forms and sizes. How do you deal with fear in your life? Do you let it easily win? Or do you use it to refine your choices and use your personal power to arrive at the right decision for you?

Is finding and following your passion the thing you most fear? Or are your thoughts more along the lines of, 'I could do anything, if only I knew what it was' (which, incidentally, is the title of a book by Barbara Sher and Barbara Smith). This book is well worth reading if you feel you lack direction regarding making your passion work for you – or if you don't even know where your true passion lies.

If you have too many conflicting passions it can be difficult to decide between them. This can result in a huge 'stuckness'. Not moving forward; standing still and sometimes sinking in quicksand. It is not healthy to experience inner conflict for too long. What is your conflict? Could it be about your work or is something else blocking the view for you to clearly see a future led by your heart and your passion?

It's important that you take some time out; to be with yourself in order to reflect on your inner desires or to read a book that discusses these areas. It might be one of the two I have mentioned here. It may be that you just need to remove yourself from 'digital land' and other people for a short time. If possible, aim to be by yourself for a few days to write and explore your passion, purpose and the next bold steps you are going to take toward to reach your dream.

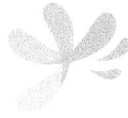

Chapter 20
Your Values and Passion

If you have been questioning the quality of your work, and your real purpose and passion in life, the following activities may help you to work out a way forward – or at least help you to understand what you really want. Or maybe it is not your work and career that is your primary concern. Maybe it is all about your life outside work – your lack of hobbies, interests or recreation in life.

Define your Values

Defining your values and finding your passion go hand-in-hand. Values are how you think and act in your life; they determine how you live your life. Your values can include what is important about your work, health, relationships with other people, what you enjoy, and what you aspire to. They determine the way you approach your life or the way you want to be in the world, and they often determine your priorities. For example, my core values are courage, honesty, generosity, creativity and adventure. These values help form how I work in the world, what I do, and how I incorporate such traits as adventure and creativity into all parts of my life.

To help you identify your values you can ask yourself the following few questions:

- When were you the happiest in life? What were you doing? What contributed to your happiness and how did it feel?

- When did you feel the most fulfilled and satisfied in your life? How and why did the experience give your life meaning?

- Was there a particular time in your past when everything seemed to fall into place? What were you doing at that time (both within your work and life in general)?

All these questions will provide you with clues and help you to uncover what your values are.

List your Values

Make a list of your values. Now choose your top ten values; then choose your top five. Following this process doesn't mean you eliminate all of your other values; it simply means that you are prioritising the top ones so you can use them to help you match your values with your life decisions. Keep a record of the other values where you can locate them at another time.

Sit with your 'big five' values for a while. Do these values feel right for you? Do they make you feel good about yourself? How would you feel if someone asked you what your values were and you told them these attributes? Try this with a good friend. Ask them if they can see these values in you.

When the things that you do in life match your values, then life usually turns out well. When you are living and doing things in life that are at odds with your values, life is usually not good. We all have values whether we identify them or not. When we identify them, we are more in tune with them and aware that when we are going against our integrity and authenticity. Use these values to make decisions and to guide what you do, and how you live.

Record your Passions

Write down what you are passionate about and what doesn't thrill or excite you.

Brainstorm everything in your life, as well as work related ideas. Don't limit yourself; just play with the ideas and let them flow. Do this quickly without thinking too much. Keep doing it until you totally exhaust everything on your list.

Here is an example of a few of my passions and areas that I'm not interested in to get you started:

I love	I am not interested in
Being creative	administration
The idea of working for myself	Managing people
Being active	Working 9–5
Freedom	Working in a big corporation

Once you have finished listing everything you can think of at the present moment, circle the top five things you love. Write them down on a separate piece of paper and then review them carefully in your mind. Are there one or two things you have always dreamed of doing in your life but didn't think you would be able to make any money doing? Or were you too scared to step outside the box? Did you just think that you were being silly and day dreaming? Maybe it frightens you to even think about them. Whatever is going through your mind, just keep playing as though this is a game and not a test or something you have to follow through with.

When you are working on the big things in your life, you could do some journaling or mind-mapping or make a list. Once you've finished, go outside into the garden to rake some leaves, cut some branches, or do some weeding. Put your hands in the soil and walk around not thinking much – just listening and doing. This activity of being in the outdoors is so enlivening and helps to resolve many challenges.

Immersing yourself in the outdoors and in your surroundings allows thoughts of self love and freedom to bubble up within you. You start to gain some clarity, bit by bit. You could even dedicate a whole weekend to work through an idea in this way. It is a great combination to work with and, like anything, as you do more of this you will build the 'muscle' of creative thinking and problem solving.

Charting your New Direction

Here are some ideas to help you to hone in on what is bubbling up for you so that you can chart your new direction:

- After you have been for a walk outside in the garden or a nearby park, your mind should be receptive for taking the next step. Sit down with your five top passions, ideas, or things that interest you. At this point, try to turn off the 'what if' analysis that happens in your mind and just keep playing.

- Get a clean sheet of paper or open up a blank Word document on your computer – whatever works best for you.

- Write down your five passions on the page. Look at them and sort them out again. Circle the top three and put the others aside. The top three should be the ones that come straight from your heart, not your head. They will be the things you would do if you had permission (from yourself or others) to do them, and nothing stood in your way.

- Take your top three passions and study them further. Now, remove one that is less important.

- Get two pieces of blank paper. Write by hand you two top passions – one on each piece of paper in large bold handwriting.

- Put them on the floor with the words facing up. Set them standing width apart. Take off your shoes. Look at them again with the love you feel for them. Then stand on them, one foot on each. Close your eyes and then go deep within in your thoughts to examine them until one of them jumps out, or quietly says 'pick me'. Step off when you know and pick up the one that resonates most strongly with you.

- This is the passion you are going to develop so that it has a greater role in your life. It might be that you will develop an idea in your spare time (which you will have to create space for in your already busy schedule). You will flesh out what you can do with this passion either as a hobby, part or full-time business, further study, a shift in your current skill-set, or perhaps even a new job. If you change your mind, that is fine too. Just trust yourself to find the answer and to find your real passion to pursue.

- You can look into ways of making this happen in your life. Do a mind-map to get the ideas out of your head and onto the page.

- Dedicate some time (at least half an hour a day) to think, write, or make plans about your new direction. If it is a new job you are seeking, you will need to make time to look for and apply for jobs. If it is transitioning from a job to your own business, you will need to explore ways to learn about business and move into a new network of business owners. If it is a hobby that could become a business in the future, work out how to get started and do it.

- Write down what the end prize would be if you were to do this thing. What will you get from doing this? How will you feel once it is underway? Pin this on the wall and remind yourself that this is what you want to achieve.

- Get yourself an accountability buddy who you can call or email to get some encouragement or 'hurry up' for those times when you fall off the wagon.

- Tell friends and family who you can trust about what you are considering. This will help you to stay on track.

- Make a pledge to yourself. Ask yourself, 'What is the worst thing that could happen if you do this?'

- Remember to take small steps – nothing ventured, nothing gained. And remember also why you are here in this life – to find your true purpose and meaning.

PART SIX

Your Relationships

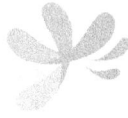

Chapter 21

How Relationships Affect Your Health and Wellbeing

"I DEFINE CONNECTION AS THE ENERGY THAT EXISTS BETWEEN PEOPLE WHEN THEY FEEL SEEN, HEARD, AND VALUED. WHEN THEY CAN GIVE AND RECEIVE WITHOUT JUDGMENT, AND WHEN THEY DERIVE SUBSTANCE AND STRENGTH FROM THE RELATIONSHIP."

- BRENÉ BROWN

In this chapter, I will share with you some of the ways that relationships can have a profound impact on your health and wellbeing, and offer some gentle ways of dealing with problematic ones. To add clarity, I have grouped all of them under three broad categories: toxic relationships, excess baggage relationships, and good to great relationships that nourish us.

Research in this field demonstrates that both the quality and quantity of our social relationships influence our mental health, physical health and mortality risk. They have an impact on our health both in the short term and long term, and these effects start in childhood and cascade throughout our lives.[20]

I know the idea of dealing with relationships can be frightening or challenging: we all prefer to avoid it with the hope that something external will produce change for us. You have to relinquish this idea; instead finding courage and thoughtfulness within to go forward and consider how to best deal with what is in front of you. Depending on your situation, you might want to 'dip your toe into the water' by starting with those relationship issues that are easiest for you to sort out. This way you will build your confidence and knowledge.

Toxic Relationships That Bring Us Down

Relationships that are toxic or troubled, and no longer nourishing will definitely have a negative impact on your health to some degree, depending on the type of relationship. According to clinical pastoral counsellor Harville Hendrix (PhD), the relationships that influence our health the most are those with our significant partner and our family.[21] I would add that some relationships within the workplace can also be very significant in terms of our psychological wellbeing, for example, those that might involve bullying or some other serious issue.

I am sure you have witnessed many women who strive to fix all aspects of their health except their relationship issues, such as a worn-out marriage, a long-term problem with a sibling, a formerly wonderful friend who no longer is, or a toxic scenario at work. This is where the hard work needs to be done to end, change or release toxic relationships in our lives. In order to improve the quality of relationships in your life, you need to give them consideration and action. Getting help from someone you trust is always a good option.

Tackling even the smallest of concerns with significant people can create fear, stress and sleeplessness. But what is the cost of not dealing with the problem? It's huge. Remember that stress and anxiety are major contributors to poor health and disease. We all carry around with us the fear of what to do about a problematic relationship; it can grind us down and sap our confidence and change us. Likewise, it can lead us to put a chain around our hearts and throw away the key. It can bring out the worst in us and sometimes the worst lingers and becomes a more entrenched part of who we are. Finally, it can make us socially withdrawn, sad and depressed.

The longer we put up with a toxic relationship with a significant person in our lives, the more entrenched our misery becomes. In the end, we can become ill and then we are forced to deal with a much more complicated situation.

We often find excuse after excuse to avoid having to confront problems in our intimate relationships, such as: 'no marriages are really happy', 'everyone is making do', or 'if I leave this marriage, I will be all alone and that is worse than staying', 'the thought of leaving is so great, I cannot bear to deal with it', and on and on it goes. If we hold onto them for a long time, nothing will change unless the relationship changes, we change our attitude towards that relationship, or we move on from it.

People who internalise troubling issues without talking to someone else or taking steps to alleviate the problems suffer quietly – but they do suffer. People who seek help from a friend, counselor or others are taking some action to resolving the relationship problem. Those who approach the issues in their relationships with courage and thoughtfulness usually find a way through that is right for them.

Harville Hendrix is known internationally for his work with couples and helping them to rectify problems within their relationship. He says that negativity is something we need to remove from our lives. He maintains that it is toxic and that once we are able to let go of it, our body will start to heal and will continue doing so. When we are free from negativity, we can substitute gratitude in its place and then we will become happy.[22]

If you are in a relationship where you or your partner are creating a lot of negativity and, worse still, if it has been there for a long period, you may need a break from each other for a while to gain sufficient clarity as to how best to deal with the problem. Staying too close to it will make it difficult to think clearly and to identify the root cause. Where relationships are concerned, clarity is one of the greatest tools available to you. Most of the inner work is achieved when you become clear and, when you reach this point, a decision is not so difficult.

Another type of relationship which can cause havoc in life is with an ex-partner with whom you share parenting of your children. Difficult divorces or separations can leave major scars if you aren't able to work out a way through it either together or for yourself.

Baggage Relationships We Can Do Without

Baggage relationships might include friendships which we once treasured but have now soured. It might be that your values are now different, or one of you is more invested than the other. Maybe someone has hurt you a few times and you now realise you no longer want that in your life.

Baggage relationships don't create the same amount of stress for us that toxic relationships do, but they do niggle at us. We examine them over and over, rationalise them and often end up doing nothing. The truth is, some friendships are not designed to last forever; many of them have a purpose and then become redundant.

When dealing with heavy relationships your values can get mixed up and you may not realises they do not nourish you. Sometimes you are even unaware of how much anxiety they cause. Letting people go is not necessarily a one-way benefit. Both of you may well be better off if you are able to break off the friendship. If you take the first step, you may actually be helping the other person as well.

If you don't weed out these types of relationships they will hinder your life and your ability to connect with people who are more suited to where and who you are at present.

We also have relationships where others rely on us for help. They may be a family member, a friend, or someone we have just met. This is fine as long as we are aware of the boundaries of our ability to help, and make sure we protect ourselves and respect the other person's point of view.

Listening is now a rare thing in our world, yet it is the most important thing we can do for each other. As a health coach, listening and asking the right questions are my top skills which help my clients create their own solutions and find clarity. Listening is key to all of your relationships. If you become a better listener, many things will change for the better in your life.

Good or Great Relationships that Nourish us

Good or great relationships usually come to us when our values are aligned in some way and we have built the relationship as a result of sharing enjoyable activities together such as travel, recreation or some other pursuit. I have a small embroidered travel pillow that one of my oldest friends gave me many years ago. I treasure this little item because it says 'The best friends are old friends', and she is my oldest friend.

Having great relationships with everyone in our lives is not very common. There are those rare people who seem to have completely harmonious connections, but the majority of us usually experience a range of different relationships, including difficult ones. Getting help from an external source such as a trusted friend or from a professional such as counsellor or psychologist is one of the best ways to resolve your relationship challenges. Generally speaking, the work involved usually centres on ourselves as well.

Defining what constitutes a great relationship is different for each of us and can often depend on being like minded. In reverse, I have often felt that the best lessons in life have come from the people we clash with or who appear to be opposed to us in some way. They often appear to teach us something about ourselves and open our minds to something new.

Great relationships occur in our life when we know who we are, what our values are, and what kind of people we want in our lives. They also come when we deal with our limiting beliefs, about ourselves or others, that we'd adopted as children and have never properly dealt with. Unfortunately, it often takes us most of our life to figure it all out.

Committing yourself to creating health in all areas of your life provides you with the wisdom of experience and space to work on your relationships. It sets you up to tackle your relationship challenges and resolve any issues.

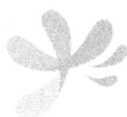

DEALING WITH CONFLICT IN FAMILY RELATIONSHIPS – MARGIE'S STORY

Margie is a successful ecological grazier and business woman, yet she has struggled with conflict in her relationships. One of the biggest challenges has been her relationship with her three brothers, who she was in partnership with in two cattle properties for many years. One was the family property where the siblings all grew up together; the other was another property that Margie drew in a ballot. Margie ran the second property while her three brothers furthered their education in order to become professionals away from the grazing life.

When it finally came time to consider dissolving the partnership between the four siblings, there were big financial issues that shocked Margie. She'd thought her brothers would acknowledge her major input into the cattle properties, whereas, instead, they saw that each of their value was equal to hers, in spite of the fact that they had largely been absent from the properties for many year.

The situation within the family escalated into legal challenges and became quite ugly. As a result, Margie's health began to decline. She could not sleep and became quite depressed. She was forced to think carefully about the situation and the outcome she wanted. She loved her property and her family, and did not want to lose either. Margie realised that she had to change her own mindset in order to extract herself from a deep dark hole.

The answer for her was a meditation retreat where she was able to calm her thoughts and learn how to retrain her mind using positive affirmations. She knew that she had to get her emotions under control; however, this was challenging and it took her time but eventually it worked. She detached herself from the property and was prepared to lose it, as well as lose her brothers.

Today, Margie still has her property and shares it with one brother and his three beautiful boys. She is grateful to have the involvement of her brother's children given she has none of her own. She is also grateful for what she does have, rather than feeling regretful for the things she does not have. She now knows success in life is not what you get out of it, but how you deal with what happens to you. Having gratitude and forgiveness played a big part in Margie's new-found peace and wellbeing.

Feeling more confident in dealing with her relationships, Margie went on to examine her relationship with her husband whom she had married later in life. She felt that as two independent people they always seemed to be competing for power, airspace, time and other things. In time, Margie realised that if she took the initiative and just loved him unconditionally, their relationship might improve. It worked and most of the big areas of conflict between her and her husband have faded away. She says they still have their differences, but she now considers their relationship to be fabulous.

Actions you can take to Improve your Relationships

Here are some actions you can take to improve the quality of your relationships:

1. It doesn't matter what the nature of a relationship is, what is important is to become aware of its impact upon you. Depending on your circumstances, you could either delve deep into your own thoughts, reflect or contemplate a course of action in the same way that Margie did, or you can seek help from a trained professional. The important thing is to not get trapped in a cyclical set of emotions that creates stress or worry, and has a negative impact on your life. Find a way to move forward, even if it is only micro steps to begin with. Acknowledge it and make a start.

2. Increase your understanding of relationships through reading either online or by finding a great book that discusses your situation. For more information, consult my further reading section at the back of this book.

3. Write a letter to someone who has hurt you. You may not send it, but the act of writing it can help to give you clarity about what to do in terms of your emotions and actions.

4. Talk to a trusted friend about your relationship. Perhaps you don't need their advice, but find it helpful to have someone who can listen and ask you questions that allow you to gain clarity.

5. If the situation is serious, find a trusted professional or family member to talk to about the problem in detail.

6. Find a way to talk to the person you are having difficulties with. If it is a work-related problem, seek advice on the best way to do this or have someone else with you if the matter is serious. If it is a friend or family member you are finding challenging to deal with, try to talk to them about what you would like to achieve rather than what you think they have done to you. Be neutral in your stance and show a willingness to resolve a problem or situation.

7. Go into nature in order to contemplate the relationship and seek clarity. Write or say affirmations that help you to focus your thoughts on resolution.

8. Seek out a meditation retreat where you can shift your perspective and potentially change the relationship as a consequence of doing inner work on yourself.

Sometimes, you will arrive at a point where the best course of action is to let go of that relationship. It is helpful if you can do this when you are clear that your life (and possibly theirs) will be better off if the relationship comes to an end.

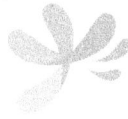

Chapter 22
Changing Negative Relationships

In the previous chapter, I discussed how relationships affect your health and wellbeing. Now we are going to gently drill down to consider all of your significant relationships and how they do or don't nourish you. I call this a relationship audit.

The purpose of doing a relationship audit is to bring to your attention what you are already aware of but may not have wanted to look closely at. You don't have to review all of your relationships at once. The idea is to take small, achievable steps in order to identify those that work and those that don't. Don't jump ahead with negative thoughts about 'what if ' or 'I feel terrible'. It is best to simply treat it as an experiment and see what happens when you do it.

Get started on your Relationship Audit

Prepare either a handwritten or digital table similar to the relationship audit table overleaf. You might also like to have your journal handy to write in if that works better for you. You might also want to define what 'nourishing' and 'not working' mean for you so that you are really clear about why you would view them in any one category.

I believe we all know what is nourishing us, but shining a light on it by undertaking this activity brings it fully to our attention and makes our understanding really clear. This doesn't mean that you are going to throw away all of the people in your life who are not nourishing you. Rather, it means that you are going to examine what is going on with these relationships and decide what kind of action you might choose to take.

For example, let's say that you have ten good friends and with two of them, the relationship seems to be a bit one way. It might be that you are the one doing all of the work to connect or vice versa. This might tell you that there is not much value in this relationship as it is.

A more difficult example may involve looking at your relationships with your siblings and parents: they may be nourishing sometimes, but not always, particularly when they are 'pressing your buttons'. These situations are easy to identify but often tricky to resolve.

You may need to examine your part in family relationships, as well as theirs. Try not to over-analyse; instead, simply write down what immediately comes to mind. There is a fair chance you have lived with your emotions related to someone in your family for some time. Maybe they neglected you some time ago and you haven't been able to forgive them and release yourself from the hurt. Maybe they just have a way of bringing out the worst in you. It might be that your first step is to protect yourself from being hurt by them. You could also write them a letter – not necessarily with the intention of posting it but to simply get things off your chest. You might also acknowledge your part in the problem in this letter. If you do this, try to step back from your emotional reactions and look at the situation without judgment.

It is important to remember that negativity is a toxin that adversely influences your physical, emotional, and mental health. The longer you put off dealing with a troubled relationship, the more your health will suffer and things will deteriorate between you and the other person. Never underestimate the impact that so-called less important relationships can have on you as well. Your logical mind may not be able to see it, but there may be some deep emotional investment in a relationship that has hurt you in the past.

Before attempting to tackle the difficult aspects of any relationship be mindful of your emotions. Putting your thoughts down on paper might bring up strong emotions and pain within you. Remember that what you feel is happening is only one part of the story – it tells you how we feel. There is another side to the story – that of the other person. So try not to judge yourself.

Relationship Audit Table

People	Nourishing/good	Neutral	Not working/ problematic	Notes
Five close friends				
Ten acquaintances				
Siblings/parents				
Intimate partner				
Work supervisor				
People you supervise				
People who influence you				

Feel free to write as much as you want in the notes or in a separate journal that is for your eyes only. It is enough to just write and contemplate what you have noticed and recorded. Awareness is the biggest part of your journey to healing your health and creating a fantastic and productive life. After awareness comes clarity and after clarity comes the ability to make a decision. Once you are in a position to make a decision, you usually act and then things change for the better. Sometimes this process is slow, while other times it can be fast. It all depends on your circumstances and your own resilience and ability to find the solution that works for you.

You may wish to examine just a couple of these relationship categories and that is fine also. It is best to take it step by step. You also may be surprised that after doing this, it seems very normal to take action to release the energy you have put into something that has not been good for you.

Protecting Yourself

The ability to properly protect yourself emotionally is an essential skill for all relationships. Why? It's a bit like Iron Man or Super Woman: you need to wear a protective shield for lots of situations when you go out in the world. Some people feed off other people's energy; some people like to put you down because of their own insecurities. If you leave yourself open, you are vulnerable to being invaded and controlled. You leave yourself open to being hurt and damaged, and then you find yourself powerless. You need to remember that you are worthy of better. You need to put yourself first, pull your emotional energy in close to you and not wear your heart on your sleeve.

Don't open yourself up to someone else's anxieties and perhaps their unconscious tendencies to hurt others. Remember, you cannot be hurt unless you allow it to occur. Once you protect yourself against others hurting or draining you, you will understand the situation better, and possibly forgive. Think of your protective shield as being similar to a super hero – they value who they are and what they are here to do in life. Release and move on from people who are unconsciously (or consciously) trying to harm you mentally, emotionally or physically. Seek professional help if the matter is serious.

A great friend of mine gave me some good advice about how to understand the majority of people in the world. She described human consciousness as being like a progression – in the same way that a child advances from kindergarten to the final year of school. Some people are in Grade one, others are in Grade five, and some are in Grade 10 or 12. Recognising this will help you have compassion for where others are in terms of their level of consciousness, and will influence your ability to grow, and wisely see things as they are. You will be able to accept people as they are, emotionally detaching from wanting them to be something they are not.

I had always found it difficult to understand why people couldn't see what I thought was so obvious. What is so simple and straight forward for us can often be difficult for someone else. The more we can learn and understand about ourselves, the more we can understand others. I do think this is the key to having great relationships: first know yourself, then know others. Knowing yourself often takes courage, and the ability to look at your parents and your siblings and shine a light on how you have been shaped through your genetics and your childhood environment. If you do the work on yourself, you will have better relationships with the people around you. In this way, you can discover those relationships that work for you.

Establishing Boundaries

Establishing boundaries is something we hear and say a lot; yet doing it properly is quite a skill. Boundaries help us to prevent things getting out of hand in relationships. People actually like to have clear boundaries imposed; it tells them how far they can go with you and where to stop. It also clarifies expectations. For example, think about dating and romantic relationships. This is one area in your life where you want to establish clear boundaries and to identify expectations. Getting the desired result when you set boundaries also depends on how you create them. Having clarity helps, as does thinking about the eventual outcome for both of you.

In order to create clear boundaries you need to prepare yourself well in advance and work out what your boundaries are with different people. Before you go into a workplace where you might have a habit of getting lost in someone else's power, quickly put your attention on how you could prevent that from happening. Review your past experiences where this might have happened to you. Think about how you could have dealt with the situation to create a different outcome. Work with this as a starting point to establishing your new boundaries. When you put your attention on something, it enables you to act on it. Without boundaries, you can get lost in other people's advice, energy and actions.

Recently, I found I was permitting too many health websites to contact me with information. I became overwhelmed and lost my clarity and focus. So I deleted most of them and drew my energy back in, and everything changed. We hold the key to how the world treats us. Use self-protection and boundaries to gain the power and clarity you need to be respected and to thrive.

Giving and Helping Others

Today we recognise that happiness or contentment comes when we are generous and give to others. We need a good measure of both giving and receiving in our lives, and there is so much capacity within us to give on so many different levels. How do you give to people in your life: to strangers, your neighbours, to work colleagues and to the world? Decide how you want to give to others and hold yourself accountable to that. Start off small and build up, then see how you feel. You should feel expanded and filled with more energy as a result.

PART SEVEN

Reflecting on Your
New Life

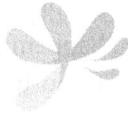

Chapter 23
Reviewing Your Progress

By choosing to do the necessary work in all of the five areas of your life – nutrition, exercise, mind, spirit, work and relationships – you will equip yourself with your own personal health blueprint for life. This journey is one of self-discovery that will power your life in the way that no other external stimulus, advice, or input will.

Each of the Five Principles of Integrative Health outlined in this book work together as an interconnected system to give you the personal power and resilience you need to create the life you desire. They are the highways of your life where you will develop and sustain high energy levels and a body that feels beautiful inside and out. You will have a life full of purpose and confidence, love and joy, and the kind of productivity that makes you wake up in the morning feeling alive knowing that this is your day and great things are happening for you. Over time, you will also be amazed by the fact that you have taken steps and have now disease-proofed your life from stress and lifestyle diseases.

As you progress on this journey to improved health and wellbeing, the ups and downs will be far less in your life and your confidence will grow. As you heal and look after all areas of your being and your inner microbiome, you will observe gradual changes. Sometimes these changes will be subtle, such as the receding of aches and pains, or the fact that your sleep is better, or that you feel calm more often.

Remember to be gentle and easy on yourself. If you take this process at a relaxed pace you will be more likely to incorporate the changes with ease and each new step will feel logical and something that you can readily do.

It may be that you are already on the journey and that this book just equips you with a few more details and things to consider. That's great and, in fact, wherever you are at this stage is commendable. The point is to get the ball rolling and to make a start.

Within my life I had a big jolt and, through necessity, had to face a whole lot of changes at once. I have found that since that deep dive I am continually learning, experimenting, and renewing my interest and approach to my own health. This is how I chose to live my life – not as if it were my religion but rather as an extremely valuable investment.

One of the most important ways to prevent yourself from going back to old habits is to keep track of your progress by recording your changes. Recording your changes spurs you on to make even more changes that reveal the benefits of who you are becoming. To do this is an investment in your ultimate wellbeing. It is also exciting to celebrate your wins. Make sure to mark these moments in your life and share them with those people who support and love you.

Use this list of helpful strategies to guide you with making improvements in your health and your life:

- Increasing my consumption of vegetables and decreasing sugar and processed foods

- Drinking more clean water; sufficient for my body to stay well hydrated

- Setting up my plate portions for what suits my body

- Checking my digestive health through tests for food sensitivities, leaky gut, candida, and thyroid health

- Excluding certain foods and increasing others

- Experimenting with different food types or diets such as bone broth, raw food, Paleo, vegan, fermented foods and others

- Increasing and sustaining my energy levels

- Knowing what my body thrives on and giving it those things

- Understanding what my cravings mean and balancing my diet according to them

- Achieving my normal weight and keeping it there

- Having more fun

- Finding a way of eating that works for me (for example, the 80/20 principle)

- Discovering a mode of exercise that suits me

- Removing devices from my bedroom at night

- Getting the right amount of sleep regularly

- Feeding my spirit through meditation, yoga, walking, nature, travel or other similar activities

- Finding my intuition and using and honing it

- Reducing chemicals in my life, including those found in cosmetics, soaps and home cleaning products

- Evaluating my relationships and making decisions about how to act on some of them

- Identifying and addressing stress in my life

- Reviewing my work and making a plan to diversify

- Exercising my mind with new ideas, concepts, and ways of doing things, as well as being open to learning new things

- Developing my awareness of negative and positive thoughts and what my habitual thinking patterns are

- Making choices to change those things I don't like and increasing those I do like

- Sticking to my goals and acknowledging or celebrating when I reach them.

Initially, work with those areas of your life that are most important to you. Use the survey from Chapter 3 to guide you and then incorporate the other aspects in later. You will discover that your interest in health will be a continual work in progress.

Here are some additional things for you to consider on your path to improved health and wellbeing:

- Can you see how integrative health can open up your life to possibilities you only ever dreamed of?

- Can you imagine living to the age of 110, functioning fully and feeling well right up until the end of your life? Would this be of interest you?

- Can you see yourself learning your entire life? Being willing to take on new projects and discovering more and more about the things that interest you?

- Can you envision a life in which you will not grow old and be a burden to others? Can you see that you will be valued because you have energy and vitality, and because you have lived well and made great choices in your life?

- Can you see yourself surrounded by a strong network of people who value their health and the impact it has on their happiness and productivity.

- Can you see a community, country, even a world where, instead of disease, we are thriving and living long and productive lives?

- Can you envision the end of chronic illnesses in society?

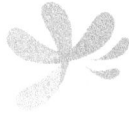

Chapter 24
Overcoming Resistance

In this chapter, I will be suggesting ways to help you when you lose your focus, become tired, and want to give up on the important things in your life.

Resistance is one of your main obstacles to having and maintaining a healthy and productive life. Resistance is the mode we default to when we find a reason not to do what we want to do. It's energising when you feel really inspired and upbeat about the future. However, I want you to also be prepared for resistance when it comes your way. It always comes to us because it is part of being human. But if you know what and how it plays out in your life, you will be two steps ahead.

The scenario goes like this: tomorrow comes and something inside you has made you flatten out a bit. You might be experiencing a nagging feeling that you can't really follow the plan you have put together; it's just too ambitious. Maybe some fear has crept in and is telling you that it's better to keep your head down and just make some minor improvements in your life. Maybe you just feel a bit uncomfortable about something and, before you know it, some doubts have crept in about your health and life ever changing.

I could go on about all of the things that can crop up and create doubt about what you are embarking upon. I am very familiar with these thoughts and I bet you are too. They can be the downfall of any great opportunity. Personally, I still have to deal with laziness as my form of resistance. It is a way of slowing me down; however, since learning about resistance, I am now much more aware of it and I can do things to avoid it. Resistance is going to play out in your life whether you like it or not. So it is a great time for you to learn about it.

The person on the planet who writes best about resistance and can help you overcome this problem is Steven Pressfield. Reading his book titled, *Do the work* changed my life.[23] According to Steven, we all experience resistance in our lives. In his book, he explains how to know it, face it and move on from it. As a result of reading Steve's book I finally understood all of the ways in which I resist doing what I want to do. I found out that the resistance within me was so sneaky that I'd never recognised that it was affecting me.

A few years ago, I was an active visual artist and my work had a lot of promise. My tutor said I was an eager student because I didn't fear failure. Then something happened to me and I became more self-aware when I was painting. Fear crept in to tell me I wasn't good enough to be a successful artist. So I gave up. I slunk away and just painted now and then. Up until that time, painting had been my greatest love and I let it go for ten years. What happened to me? Where had the joy I felt when I started working on a new canvas gone? A form of resistance entered me, masquerading as rationality. I believed I was not good enough and that was the sad end of my painting career.

Pressfield's book helps you to recognise all the tricks of your resistant mind, and how to deal with them when they: attempt to make you give up on something, tell you you're not good enough, or constantly distract you from getting on with things. You will learn to know your resistant traits, and how they stop you from achieving what is important.

I recommend that you obtain a copy of his book and read it thoroughly. It will change your life, and if it doesn't, it is probably resistance telling you not to get too excited about overcoming resistance. Just do it. Keep the knowledge first and foremost in your mind. Be the warrior in your life and be protective of what you are creating.

Steven Pressfield's book *Do the Work* is highly recommended and his other books are worth a look too. He has a number of business books and novels which can be found on Amazon. If you would like to learn more about the author and his books you can find him online at www.stevenpressfield.com.

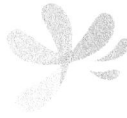

Chapter 25
A New Vision

A vision statement – whether it is written in words, drawn in pictures or recorded on your phone – is a view or map to guide your dreams and desires, and it is more than simply a handy thing to have. A vision is a code that guides your life in the direction you want to go. All successful people have some kind of vision of the direction they want their lives to take. When you create a vision with a powerful intent, your subconscious mind records your desire and helps you to stay on the path towards the end point. Often, the end point of one vision is the start for the next vision you might have for your life.

Developing a Vision for your Life

Once you have made the effort to discover your values, as well as your key strengths and weaknesses, the next step is to develop a vision for your life.

A vision statement can be asserted as if you are already living it. For example, here is a simple vision statement: I created for my own life: *'My life is filled with energy and vitality. I have a successful business I love, I have built a great community around health, and I help women all over the world regain their health. I live in the country and grow most of my food. My life is well adjusted for work and pleasure. I spend three months of each year travelling and writing. I am the happiest and healthiest I have ever been'.* Approximately fifty words is an ideal length for a vision statement. You don't want it to be too long or too short in order to really paint the picture of your life.

So it's time to get started with pen and paper and start jotting down ideas for your vision statement or making a vision board. Don't aim for 100 per cent clarity or perfection; just play around with your thoughts and ideas that you may have had for some time and try a few out.

You could think about the important aspects of your life such as health, career, lifestyle, travel, relationships, family, financial matters, education or anything else that is important to your life. At this stage, you don't want to get bogged down with micro details. A vision is a big picture of your life. Think about what you would like people to say about you after you have gone from your life. Who were you? What things have defined your life? Answering these questions can help you to form a vision for your life going forward. What actions do you undertake in your life? Write these things down and then reverse that concept into a forward vision.

For example, you might be a person who helps children become healthy, or you may be someone who helps elderly people have good quality of life in their later years. Or perhaps you are a writer or an artist who achieves certain accolades in your artistic field. Or your vision might be more connected to family and having the people you love around you. Or it could be to live self-sufficiently and grow your own food. Whatever it is, it is your vision, not someone else's.

Once you have completed your vision statement or board, put it aside so that you can come back to revisit it later.

Set Goals to Move in the Right Direction

In Chapter 2, I discussed the importance of setting your personal goals before embarking on your journey to improved health and wellbeing. It is a good idea to regularly review your goals and make any necessary changes as you go through life. At this point, you might want to make some long-term goals – even up to 20 years ahead can be fun and interesting to plan out in advance. Long-term goals are usually less detailed than short-term ones because it is hard to provide details for something that is in the distant future.

Remember, goals hold you to your dreams and provide you with the action steps to make them happen. Often we find that ten years have gone by and we still haven't done the thing we most wanted to do. Think about all those things you currently want or have wanted in the past but have never done. These could be your goals that fit in with your vision which, in turn, align with your values and your strengths.

By now you will probably be feeling a sense of lightness and excitement about how you can take your life forward. You will have developed a new self-awareness and a precious insight into who you really are and what you need to do to create the best life possible for yourself.

At this point, it is time to make a commitment to your life. Do you truly want the best life you can have? Not what others think is appropriate for you but what you really want for yourself?

Your Mission Statement for your Best Life

There is one final important thing left for you to do – to create your mission statement for each of your goals

Here is a suggested procedure for establishing your mission statement for your life goals:

- Think about all of your current goals and have them in mind for this exercise.

- Get a clean sheet of paper. The question you need to ask yourself is: 'How do I achieve the goals I have created?' You need to develop a mission statement for each goal which tells you how you will reach it. For example, you might be asking how you can enter into your new career? Or how do you save enough money to travel every year? Or how you can afford to buy some land so you can be self-sufficient?

- Divide the page into four squares. At the top of each square, write one of four goals; place a goal in each quadrant.

- Think up about four 'how to get there' statements for each goal. For example, in order to have sufficient funds to travel overseas each year, you might be able to tighten your budget to save 10-15 per cent more to cover costs on top of your travel funds for airfares and accommodation. That would be one 'how to' point. Continue on until you finish the exercise for the four goals.

This will be your mission statement – your way forward in life. You can set it aside and go back to it to refine it or to change certain aspects. Now that you have committed your mission statement in writing, you have made it real in your life. Declaring your intent through writing down your vision, goals, and mission is the act of declaring to yourself what will happen in your life.

The tricky part of all this is to be careful what you wish for. For example, if you want to meet the man or woman of your dreams you need to be sure to include the details of what they might be like. If you want to travel in comfort, make sure you include this detail and how it could happen.

Now that you have declared what you want and how you are going to get it, you will start to see opportunities that support these actions. This isn't magic. Yet those people who don't do these exercises in their life are likely to never be aware of the opportunities that present themselves to make their dreams happen.

Sometimes your mission statement will change or take a new turn because something else wonderful has come up in your life. That is fine also because changing our minds is something the world allows us to do.

BONUS
SECTION

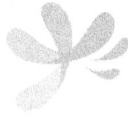

Chapter 26

How to stay Healthy when You Travel

If you are a busy high-achieving woman you probably travel quite a lot for your work. This could be to a local or international destination; to a developing country or to a developed country. In any case, it is quite likely that you will find that your normal healthy eating routine is very easily disrupted whenever you travel.

When you are in an unfamiliar environment, it can often be challenging to locate your version of healthy food, particularly if you are on a particular health regime or because you have Celiac disease, or are sensitive to gluten, dairy or other foods. You might be in the middle of a specific nutritional program such as a candida cleansing diet or a detox and then suddenly you are requested to travel interstate or overseas for your job. The thought of risking all of the hard work you have been doing to get your body back in shape can lead to other issues such as anxiety or feeling resigned to never being able to achieve your health goals.

This can be quite a complex situation, particularly if you need to get well or lose weight and your work demands that you travel frequently.

On top of this there is always the risk of getting some type of bug or intestinal problems from travel, especially if you are visiting developing countries.

The last thing any of you need is a situation which creates a lot of anxiety or stress about the health dangers of travel. I had to resolve this dilemma in my own life, so I wrote this chapter to help those of you who find yourselves in this situation.

My sister has a great attitude to life and to what she eats. Her approach is to not pay attention to the problems that can occur with travelling; rather she tends to focus on all the things that can (and do) go right. I take a lot of comfort from her relaxed outlook and it serves as a reminder to me of the importance of perspective.

It is important to recognise any self-sabotage tendencies you might have, whether they be to lose focus on what you are currently doing to benefit your health, to abandon your new healthy eating regime altogether, or to throw caution to the wind and as a result pick up a bug that you could have otherwise avoided. If your digestive system has been previously compromised, my advice is to minimise your exposure to potential pathogens without tying yourself up in knots so you don't enjoy your travel experiences.

One of the best ways to do this is to be mentally and physically prepared with some sensible strategies and actions ready to put in place during your trip.

Identify your own dietary challenges when travelling

My number one suggestion when travelling is to identify well ahead the things that can disrupt your healthy eating habits, either as a result of the physical situation you find yourself in or through abandoning of your usual healthy habits.

To help you to prepare for any unforeseen situations, I have compiled a list of some things to clarify with yourself before you travel. You might want to add some more of your own roadblocks that prevent you from sticking to your normal dietary guidelines to this list. They can be perceived things that you impose on yourself or genuine difficulties. The idea is to identify them and work out what you can (and can't) control.

Possible reasons why you might let you health go when you are travelling include:

- You have a habit of abandoning your current nutritional regime when you travel. How open are you to making the effort to plan and prepare for healthy eating while travelling?

- You have special needs for your diet which are not easily available where you travel.

- You are attending a conference, meetings or workshops and prefer not to make a fuss about your dietary requirements.

- You have a tendency to get caught up in all the other aspects of travel and consequently your dietary requirements are not a priority.

- It all seems too hard to manage your new health program while you are traveling.

Often travel does disrupt our previously established health routines. However, it's relatively simple to minimise the disruption by using a few handy things you bring with you that will help to keep you on track. And the advantage is that by making the effort, you know that you will feel all the better for it.

One of the most useful things you can do to maintain your health is to pre-plan your trip by researching where health food shops and healthy restaurants are, that serve the sort of food you want, and need are located.

Foodstuffs and other items you can take with you

Depending on how much room you have available in your baggage, you might like to take any items from the following list that suit your mode of travel and your requirements:

1. Healthy snacks for the plane trip (and beyond), especially if it is a long one. These could include nuts, dark chocolate with minimal sugar, a green apple, some chopped raw vegetables with a healthy dip, or a homemade healthy slice that you prepare and maybe freeze in advance.

2. Make sure you register your dietary requirements with the airline if they provide meals on the flight.

3. A travel blender (either electric or hand shaker) to make healthy smoothies in your hotel room.

4. Mix a bunch of smoothie ingredients in a container before you go on your trip to use as either a meal or a supplement to a meal if you get caught out or want a quick power-packed shake in the morning. This kind of smoothie will help to enhance your gut health, bowel movements, and immunity while travelling. It is a great insurance policy if you cannot find proper nutrition or functional foods in certain places and at specific times. A suggested smoothie mix includes the following high–quality ingredients:

    -   Raw green powder

    -   Pea protein powder

    -   Ground chia seeds for fibre

    -   Maca powder (the cacao flavored version is delicious)

When you arrive at your destination, pick up some low sugar fruit to mix in with it and also some coconut water. These days you can also buy concentrated coconut water. The main thing is to always check the sugar content of these items.

This form of nutrition is especially helpful if you are in and out of a conference, workshops, or meetings and need nutrients you can trust. You can make up two batches in the morning and visit your room, or take with you and consume it quickly and easily.

5. Some high-quality immune boosting teabags such as echinacha tea or powdered matcha green tea which can easily be mixed up in a cup with some hot water.

6. If you are following a gluten-free diet, take a loaf of gluten free bread with you if you want to have breakfast in the hotel.

7. Pack health supplements to keep you healthy including a high-quality general probiotic, vegetable enzymes to help out with digestive issues, Vitamin B, and some immune-boosting supplements such as vitamin C. You can also start taking them before you go and during your trip. Take any other medication you would normally take with you.

8. Those of you who are following a gluten-free diet may find a product called Glutenza very helpful. It is not simply an excuse to eat gluten but if you are concerned about cross contamination or a restaurant that isn't vigilant about gluten free items on the menu, you can take one or two tablets an hour before eating and up to 1.5 hour after eating. Glutenza contains specific enzymes that break down gluten before it gets into the lower intestines. It can be obtained online at the following Amazon link[24]: http://www.amazon.com/NuMedica-Glutenza-60-Vegetable-Capsules/dp/B00NPEYC5M

9. During a long plane trip, consume as much water as you can before and during the flight. Hydration is the key for plane travel. Don't worry about how many times you have go to the toilet – drinking lots of water will help to minimise jet lag.

10. Any special foods or supplements that you know help you when you need a 'pick-me-up'.

Ways to boost your nutrition after arriving at your destination

Once you have arrived at your destination, there are some useful things you can do to establish healthy eating patterns straight away including browsing local shops or markets or asking for advice at the hotel desk.

- Find where you can buy fresh (possibly organic) food to eat and to take away. Buy some fruit and healthy snacks to take to meetings or the event you have come for.

- Take healthy snacks such as nuts to your meetings or events so you aren't hungry when everyone else is consuming what is served up.

- Find the restaurants that suit your nutritional requirements and have the names and locations on hand when you need them. For example, if you meet some colleagues or make some new acquaintances, you can suggest a restaurant to go to.

- When eating out, choose options that are aligned with your healthy eating regime at home. If the menu doesn't offer what you want, request them to make you a similar dish. Some people don't even read the menu; they simply request a meal they want. Most places will be happy to prepare your requested dish if it is straightforward.

- Buy a stock of filtered water bottles for your hotel room to have on hand all the time.

- Remember the 80/20 rule to eat healthily most of the time and then have what you want for 20 per cent of the time. Dedicate your 20 per cent to restaurant meals if you feel like doing so.

- If you are limiting your alcohol consumption, drink water before and after a glass of alcohol.

- Remember the golden rule to crowd out the food items you don't want to go overboard on with other things that you can have.

- When you are visiting a new country, seek out local cultured foods. Every destination has different cultured foods that are local to it. Try eating it – your gut will enjoy some new healthy bacteria from another culture.

- Don't fret or worry too much about your dietary requirements. Have a great time enjoying your new experiences.

My single biggest tip for high achieving women who travel for work is to choose a couple of things that will make a difference to your ability to stick to healthy foods. Do this for your first trip and then add more things for next time. Small easy steps are the most successful way to create this method of maintaining health when travelling.

Finally, keep a list of things you particularly liked and want to add to the diversity of foods you consume when you travel. Also, keep some notes on any good ideas you get for your next trip.

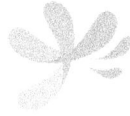

Chapter 27

How to Fit Exercise in when You Travel

This chapter complements the previous one in which I explained how to eat well when you travel for work. Both of these goals are far more important than they might initially seem to be. I recommend that you make exercising when travelling one of your health priorities. Why? Because you deserve more than having changes to your usual routine determine your health and your life.

We reach this place of health and vitality when we take small, achievable steps towards the ideal of being powered by health – an ideal that is different for each of us. Gaining and maintaining our health is initially about self-awareness and then moves on to self-discovery which involves nurturing our health, especially in areas we find challenging. As a result, we come to deeply honor who we are because we have built an intimate relationship with our bodies and our lifestyle.

If you travel frequently for work and you haven't yet worked out a way to maintain your exercise program, there are some simple things you can do regardless of how busy your schedule is. The best way to tackle this dilemma of struggling to keep exercising when you travel is to add in small strategies that you can adopt easily. Don't aim for the 'big plan' and then find you cannot achieve it. It is so much easier to do when you take small, incremental steps.

Plan your Exercise Strategy before Travelling

Before embarking on your travels, ask yourself the following questions:

- Where do you mostly travel to for work?
- What exercise do you think you will be able to incorporate in your daily schedule while you are away from home? What is the easiest form of exercise for you to actually do?
- What exercise do you currently do at home that will fit into your type of travel and the places you visit? Do you go to the gym, run, swim, walk or do something else?
- Considering your current habits and schedule, what is the most likely time for you to exercise? Is it first thing in the morning or at the end of a big day?

Remember, when you are travelling for work your free time will probably be limited so your exercise program doesn't need to be elaborate. It can simply be maintenance exercise. Think about what happens to your body when you travel and don't get enough exercise. Decide which type of exercise is most likely for you to be able to do while you are travelling. Then, start following this regime before you leave home to get into the groove of doing it when you are away. Aim small and build on your progress. Finally, make it fun.

Research Exercise Options before you go

It is always a great idea to do some research on exercise options that are available at your travel destination. Doing this will highlight options for walking, visiting interesting tourist or local areas, and ways to combine enjoyment of learning about the place you are staying at and exercising in that location.

Doing some research will also motivate you to include certain activities in your already busy schedule. As you are probably aware, if you bond with an idea and add it to your diary or schedule, you will have a far greater chance of actually doing it. Furthermore, when you do it, you will strengthen your resolve to continue doing exercise that you enjoy when you travel.

Look for gyms or yoga classes if that is your thing, or a pool in a hotel that you can book into, or an interesting place to walk to. In many parts of Asia, local parks are used for dancing, exercise, singing and all kinds of community and health-related pursuits.

The central message here is to combine local experiences with your exercise regime when you travel.

Other Exercise Options

Aim to do stretching exercises or some yoga asanas in your hotel room for 15 minutes. This is useful if you are unable to get outdoors to exercise.

You can also add a morning practice of stretching for 15 minutes before breakfast or doing any form of work. During this routine, aim to stretch every part of your body so that it sets your posture up for the rest of the day. By following this routine, along with other types of regular exercise, you will be able to keep your body in good health.

Don't make the mistake of getting stuck in your hotel room and just going out for dinner and to attend work commitments. Walk at lunch time, even if it is just a brief stroll around the block. Movement of all kind is helpful and will keep your body in good condition.

Make your exercise regime fun by teaming up with someone you are travelling with to go for an early morning walk. That way you cannot easily escape to emails and other distractions.

Some tips for dealing with the unexpected (or expected)

When you are required to travel for your career, you will find that people are always trying to attract your attention to do this or do that, or there is always an opportunity to stitch up that next deal or plant a seed with a new prospect or colleague. We are flooded with a long list of things to do, places to be, and timelines in which to get everything done.

It is my experience that by clearly defining your priorities for your work and your health, many of the daily demands take on a different meaning and can fit around your priorities. In fact, if you are a person of influence, it is up to you to demonstrate to others through your actions that doing certain things for your health is crucial for your energy levels and ability to handle busy schedules without getting run down. It is akin to brushing your teeth – it needs to happen regularly.

When you move into this space of valuing your health and your time for exercise, people, places and things bend to you a bit more and everything works out just fine.

Don't become that dreary person who abstains from mixing with other people who are drinking and eating things you may not want to personally engage in. This can happen if you don't insist on making time for your personal health priorities such as exercise. If you do attend to your health and exercise priorities, you will be more likely to want to mix socially with work or other colleagues. Plus, you will have a different attitude – maybe less resentful or grumpy – towards them because you have looked after your own needs first.

This process might initially take a bit of practice if you are used to responding to many competing issues and demands. You will need to be able to regulate your own behaviour first and then notice how things around you change to fit in with your standpoint. It works – try it for yourself. Be well prepared for your travel. Pack what you need to help you to maintain your health and take any necessary steps towards ensuring it. Don't worry if it doesn't all work out as neatly as you had originally planned. Just make a start and focus on the benefits of incorporating some exercise into your daily schedule when you travel.

NEXT STEPS

The most effective way to stay on top of your game is to have enough energy to power your life, yet this is one of the most common health problems busy women deal with.

This book is about embracing my Five Principles of Integrative Health and discovering that intimate relationship with all of you – your body, mind and spirit. I call this concept 'coming home to you'. Integrative health is about taking care of all parts of your being. You are like a multifaceted diamond – each of these facets needs to be understood and developed.

If you can apply two or three suggestions from this book and stick with them, you will begin to observe changes in your health and in your life: sometimes small, sometimes quite noticeable. From these seeds you will grow the shoots, branches and flowers of your new life. This tree will be resilient in the face of the ravages of life, because there will be no gaps or no stone unturned in your journey to true health. You will deal with every aspect of your life and you will know that by the peace you will experience.

Your body has an innate wisdom and knows how to heal itself. Once this starts to become evident to you, you will feel so much more motivated to keep going on your health journey.

What being powered by health really means

Being powered by health involves working with the Five Principles of Integrative Health that I have outlined in this book. It means being fully interconnected in these five key areas – nutrition and fitness; mindset; spiritual wellbeing; career and work; and relationships – so you are powered for a life of health, vitality and productivity.

Start with energy

Energy powers everything in life. When you have strong reserves of ongoing energy, you look and feel positive and vital.

When working with my clients, the first step involves unlocking ways in which they can improve their energy levels. This helps them to see beyond the pain they are currently experiencing in their lives. When energy is lagging, I help clients kick-start their recovery process by advising on nutrition, sleep, exercise, mindset and purpose.

This may sound overly simplistic to you but it is often the simple easy-to-fix things that we overlook. Once you have more energy, you will be able to see and think more clearly, feel more motivated and have greater momentum for undertaking your journey to better health.

With increased available energy, you can continue to experiment as you tackle all the other aspects of your health and your life. Don't put a strict time limit on achieving this goal. This is not like a diet. It's about changing old habits for new ones and the way to do this is to crowd them out so that it is easier for you to reach your goals. This book is not about strict eating regimes. Rather, it is about losing weight the healthy and sustainable way. As I mentioned in Chapter 4, my favourite way to eat is to follow the 80/20 principle. For 80 per cent of the time I eat healthy foods and for the other 20 per cent of the time, I eat whatever I want.

Over time, your taste buds and desire for food that doesn't nourish you will change. You will find yourself seeking out healthy treats and healthy food most of the time. You will have crossed the magic line in the sand where you love your new lifestyle over your old way of being. You will have reinvented yourself in your own time.

If you follow the guidelines in this book you will notice the following changes:

- Positive changes in your weight, digestion, skin tone, and eye brightness. Other people will notice and comment on how well you are looking, and it will be true. They will see you differently and want what you have.

- Your body will delight you as it finds its own natural shape and weight.

- Each small change or adjustment you make will give you more confidence and motivation.

- You will sleep well and feel much better for it. You will value your sleep and properly guard it.

- You will know what nourishes you in all areas of your life. You will increasingly exclude people, places, things, foods, and events that no longer enrich you, and where you don't do that, it will be because you have chosen not to. You will no longer be unconscious about what doesn't nourish you.

- You will have greater clarity in your life. Decisions will come much easier to you because you have travelled a path of identifying what really matters to you, and what makes you thrive.

- You will be ready for more and different possibilities for your life and you will not hesitate to engage with people who you deem as being beneficial, fun and appealing.

- Regardless of your age, you will look in the mirror and you will see yourself as beautiful. How could you not if you have spent time and energy redirecting your life to become beautiful from the inside out. You will laugh with a combination of joy and amazement about how you did this, and you will thank yourself.

- With less processed sugar in your diet, your blood sugar levels will be more even and you will have fewer highs and lows. You will flow through life with a new sense of calm.

- As you have more love for your whole self, you will have more love and compassion for others around you. You will understand and see more clearly how most of society has drifted away from looking after themselves, and the inherent disadvantages of this.

- You will go further into your being because you will develop a deeper interest in your health. You will try new things and approaches, and you will research areas that interest you.

- You will have patience because you will recognise how your body and, in turn, your life thrives when you look after your health and your life as a whole. Patience will enable you to continue on your health journey because you will become fascinated with all that you can become.

- Because you are unique, other pleasant surprises will occur that are meant for you and only you.

The Five Principles of Integrated Health outlined in this book are your insurance policy for a healthy, productive and vital life. This approach allows no opportunity for gaps or cracks to appear that disrupt your physical, mental or spiritual wellbeing. For the rest of your life, you will have your own place to call home that supports and sustains you. The love, comfort, strength, stability and knowledge you will develop will power your new wonder-filled meaningful and healthy life, full of possibilities.

REFERENCES

INTRODUCTION

1. Minich, D. (PhD), Pers Comm. A Grain of Truth Power Hour with Dr. Tom O'Bryan, 2015

PART ONE

Chapter 1

2. Moloney, RD. Desbonnet, L. Clark, G. Dinan, TG. Cryan, JF. *The Microbiome: stress, health and disease,* 2013 Springer Science+Business, Media New York, in Mamm Genome, 2014

PART TWO

Chapter 4

3. Sansouci, Jenny. 'Why cut out nightshade vegetables', in an article on Dr. Frank Lipman's Blog, retrieved on http://www.drfranklipman.com/why-cut-out-nightshade-vegetables/

Chapter 5

4. Nestle, Marion. 'Is saturated fat a problem?' in Food Politics Blog, retrieved on http://www.foodpolitics.com/2014/03/is-saturated-fat-a-problem-food-for-debate/

5. ABC Health & Wellbeing. 'Diet and saturated fat: what to believe', retrieved from http://www.abc.net.au/health/features/stories/2013/11/04/3883432.htm

6. Weil, Andrew. 'Dr. Weil's Anti-Inflammatory Diet', retrieved from http://www.drweil.com/drw/u/ART02012/anti-inflammatory-diet

7. Australian Government, Australian Institute of Health and Welfare, in online report, 'Australia's Health 2012, How much do we spend on Health?' retrieved from http://www.aihw.gov.au/australias-health/2012/spending-on-health/#c1

Chapter 7

8. 'Reboot with Joe: juicing for weight loss with Joe Cross', retrieved from http://www.rebootwithjoe.com/

Chapter 9

9. Nakayama, Andrea, Pers Comm. 'Digestive Round Table Interviews', Jason Hawrelak.

10. 'Broth of Life: Bone broth', retrieved from http://www.brothoflife.com.au

PART THREE

Chapter 12

11. Rosenthal, Joshua. *Integrative Nutrition: Feed your hunger for Health and Happiness*, New York, 2013.

Chapter 13

12. Wikipedia, the free Encyclopedia – Hebbian Theory, This commonly used phrase was first used in 1949 by Donald Hebb, a Canadian neuropsychologist who achieved a great deal in his work on associative learning. According to Hebb, every experience, thought, feeling, sensation, and even muscle action we undergo becomes embedded in the network of brain cells that, in turn, produce the events or experiences in our lives. Every time we repeat a thought or action, the connection in our brain is strengthened and is repeated in our lives.

13. Doidge, Norman. *The Brain that Changes itself*, Penguin Publishing, USA. 2007

14. Arden, John, B, (PhD). *Rewire Your Brain: Think Your Way to a Better Life*, John Wiley & Sons, New Jersey, 2010

Chapter 14

15. Cameron, Julia. *The Artist's Way: A Spiritual Path to Higher Creativity*, Penguin Group, USA, 1992

PART FOUR
Chapter 16

16. The Australian Government, Australian Institute of Health and Welfare, 2014, *Australia's Health in 2014 in Brief*, Australian Government.

Chapter 17

17. Marselle, Melissa R. Irvine, Katherine N. and Warber, Sara L., 'Examining Group Walks in Nature and Multiple Aspects of Well-being: A large-scale study', *Ecopsychology*, September 2014

18. The Huffington Post, 'The Third Metric: Taking a walk in Nature could be the best thing you do for mood all day', retrieved from http://www.huffingtonpost.com/2014/09/23/walk-nature-depression_n_5870134.html

19. Peter, HK Jnr. Patricia, HH. (editors), *The Rediscovery of the Wild*, Massachusetts Institute of Technology, 2013

PART SIX
Chapter 21

20. Umberson, D. & Karas Montez, J. *Social Relationships and Health: A Flashpoint for Health Policy*, University of Texas, 2010

21. Institute for Integrative Nutrition, Health Coaching Lectures, pers comm. Harville Hendrix (PhD).

22. Institute for Integrative Nutrition, Health Coaching Lectures, pers comm. Harville Hendrix (PhD).

Chapter 24
23. Steven, P. *Do the Work,* Do You Zoom Inc, USA, 2011

BONUS SECTION
Chapter 26
24. 'How to purchase Glutenza', retrieved from http://www.amazon.com/NuMedica-Glutenza-60-Vegetable-Capsules/dp/B00NPEYC5M

FURTHER READING

- Joshua Rosenthal, *Integrative Nutrition: Feed your hunger for Health and Happiness*, 2013.

- Julia Cameron, *The Artist's Way Every Day: A Year of Creative Living*, 1992

- Richard Louv, *The Nature Principle: Reconnecting with Nature in a Virtual Age*, 2012

- Paramhansa Yogananda, *Autobiography of a Yogi*, 1955

- Dr Linda Wilson, *Stress Made Easy: Peeling Women off the Ceiling*, 2015

- Susan Jeffers (PhD), *Feel the Fear and do it Anyway*, 1987

- Harville Hendrix (PhD), *Getting the Love You Want: A Guide for Couples*, 1988

- Harville Hendrix (PhD) and Helen Lakelly Hunt (PhD), *Making Marriage Simple*, 2013

- Clarissa Rayward, *Splitsville: How to Separate, Stay out of Court and Stay Friends*, 2014

- Steven Pressfield, *Do the Work: Overcome Resistance and Get out of Your Own Way*, 2011

- Steven Pressfield, *The War of Art: Break through your Blocks and Win your Inner Creativity*, 2002

ABOUT THE AUTHOR

SHORT

Amanda Bigelow is a certified health coach and behavior change specialist who works with high-achieving women, helping them to create abundant energy, healthy bodies and inspired, productive lives. Amanda lives in Brisbane, Australia and works with women throughout Australia and internationally. www.amandabigelow.com.

LONG

Amanda Bigelow is a certified Integrative Nutrition health coach and behavior change specialist. She holds a Bachelor of Applied Science and was awarded a Winston Churchill Fellowship for her work with Indigenous Australians.

Amanda works with high-achieving women and is passionate about helping them to create abundant energy, healthy bodies and inspired, productive lives. Drawing from her own health journey, she uses a five-step health framework that enables women to get their energy back, exercise in a way their body loves, create a powerful mindset, tap into their spiritual wellbeing, and take their life to a whole new level.

Before becoming a health coach, Amanda had a successful career as a CEO for environmental companies, and as an environmental adviser working with local communities, governments and businesses in Australia and internationally. She has supported people all around the world to build a healthier planet through restoring rivers, soil, and managing their lands sustainably.

Amanda is an experienced public speaker who draws on both her health and environmental knowledge to craft a new vision for our 21st century lives. She lectures on a range of health-related topics including: digestive health and nutrition, stress and anxiety, lifestyle diseases, sleep, and creating an inspired and energised life. She also speaks about the important role that women play in our society today and the benefits of nature for our wellbeing.

As a result of her insight and practical step-by-step method for helping women with their health challenges, Amanda is known for leaving her clients feeling that they have been supported all the way and that the journey to complete health is much simpler than they'd thought.

If you are looking for a compassionate and knowledgeable health professional who can help you to navigate the pathway from where you are today to where you dream of being, Amanda is that person.

For more information about Amanda's five-step health framework and one-on-one health consultations, visit:

www.amandabigelow.com or by email on: ab@amandabigelow.com

Notes:

Notes:

Notes: